Qigong

BA DUAN JIN

Practical Tutorials for **Health, Vitality, and Inner Harmony**

By Zhao Xiaoting

SCPG

Text by Zhao Xiaoting
Translation by Han Chouping
Cover and Interior Design by Wang Wei

Editors: Cao Yue, Yang Wenjing

ISBN: 978-1-63288-057-4

Address any comments about *Qigong: Ba Duan Jin* to:

SCPG
401 Broadway, Ste.1000
New York, NY 10013
USA

or

Shanghai Press and Publishing Development Co., Ltd.
Floor 5, No. 390 Fuzhou Road, Shanghai, China (200001)
Email: sppd@sppdbook.com

Printed in China by RR Donnelley Asia Printing Solutions Limited

1 3 5 7 9 10 8 6 4 2

Contents

Preface

Traditional Chinese health cultivation includes a variety of body-mind exercises, which are deeply rooted in ancient Chinese philosophy and medicine. Today, the concept of "health initiative (an ability to achieve physical, mental and social well-being)" has become well recognized. Traditional Chinese health cultivation exercises are attracting worldwide attention because of their unique effects in regulating the breathing, body and mind.

Traditional Chinese health cultivation has a long-standing and well-established history. As an important part of health cultivation practice, *Dao Yin* exercise was used for disease prevention and treatment as well as life cultivation before acupuncture, moxibustion and herbal medicine. The recordings of *Dao Yin* and its specific exercise methods can be traced back to the *Zhuangzi*, *LüShi ChunQiu* (*Master Lü's Spring and Autumn Annals*), *Huangdi Neijing* (*The Inner Canon of the Yellow Emperor*), and archaeologically unearthed books such as *Yin Shu* (*A Book on Dao Yin*) and *Dao Yin Tu* (*Dao Yin Diagram*). After this, the thousands of years have witnessed the enrichment, progress and innovation of Chinese *Dao Yin* practice, coupled with emergence of numerous methods and perfection of its theoretical system. In late 20th century, the ancient *Dao Yin* exercise became exceptionally popular across China in the form of *Qigong*.

Today, Chinese *Dao Yin* exercise remains flourishing with its holistic "Man-Nature Unity" idea and various exercise methods that benefit both body and mind. Facts show that there is a profound academic system behind Chinese *Dao Yin* exercise. This system studies the interactions between material foundation (essence) and self-organization ability (mind). In other words, it studies the way to achieve harmony and coordination of human being—the most complex system on earth.

This book introduces one of the modern Chinese *Dao Yin* exercises, *Ba Duan Jin*, covering its historical origin, theoretical foundation, key principles, illustrated movements, step-by-step explanations, and practical applications. It combines detailed illustrations and video footage to facilitate learning and practice for health cultivation enthusiasts.

Chapter One
History and Theoretical Foundation

Ba Duan Jin is an ancient practice that can be traced back to thousands of years ago. It consists of eight movements. The word *Jin* (literally a silken quality like a piece of brocade) means precious or valuable. According to legend, Daoist immortals practiced *Ba Duan Jin* to lay foundations for inner alchemy and eminent monks practiced *Ba Duan Jin* for *Chan (Zen)*-meditation. The common people practiced *Ba Duan Jin* to remove diseases and improve health.

History

Ba Duan Jin has a very long history of development. As the story goes, a Daoist priest in the East Jin dynasty (317–420) named Xu Xun was the patriarch of Jing Ming Daoist Branch (Pure Brightness Sect). He was also known as the legendary Sublime Saviour of Divine Virtuosity (*Shen Gong Miao Ji Zhen Jun*), and is believed to be the figure referred to in the well-known folk saying: "When a man attains the *Dao*, all his family including fowls and dogs ascend to heaven." In addition, Xu Xun was also the author of Daoism classics including *Ling Jian Zi*.

The *Ling Jian Zi Yin Dao Zi Wu Ji Yin Dao Jue* (Ling Jianzi's Record of *Dao Yin* between the Hours of *Zi* and *Wu*) states, "Two hands hold up the heaven to regulate *Sanjiao*, drawing the bow left (the liver) and right (the lung) to shoot the hawk, strengthen the liver and kidneys using two hands, hold the left elbow with the right hand and look to the left and vice versa to regulate emotions, abduce and shake two arms to benefit the heart, two hands hold the soles to strengthen the low back, and cover the ears with two hands to click teeth 36 times, and tap the postauricular bone using the index finger" (the volume 10 of the *Daozang* or *Daoist Canon*). These eight sentences summarized seven movements. Although these movements were not named as *Ba Duan Jin*, they are the early verses of *Ba Duan Jin*.

According to Xu Xun, he once learned the *Tai Shang Ling Bao Jing Ming Fa* from an immortal, including the method of fighting against dragons and killing snakes. During his official service, he had done many things to help the people. Xu Xun was already 136 years old in the second year of Ningkang era (AD 374). On the first day of the eighth lunar month of that year, his whole family of 42 persons ascended to the heaven, together with their fowls and dogs. He was venerated as Xu Immortal (*Xian*). Before ascending to the heaven, Xu Xun thrust his sword into the roof of his house. This had two purposes: one is to keep the ninth son of the dragon spraying water to suppress fire; the other is to repel demons and evil spirits. Today, Xu families in Jiangxi Province still consider Xu Xun as their guarding angel.

Tao Hongjing (456–536) is a well-known medical expert, alchemist and writer in the Southern Liang dynasty (502–557). Although he lived a secluded life in the mountains, he remained an adviser and friend to the then Emperor Wu of Liang (464–549). Consequently, Tao Hongjing had the nickname Prime Minister in the Mountains. The Emperor Wu of Liang once issued an imperial edict saying "what can the mountains offer you?" (Implying that there's nothing in the mountains and he should be a government official). Tao Hongjing wrote a poem to reply the emperor:

What can the mountains offer me?
Nothing but the clouds white and free.
Though enjoy the scene with content,
To you, my lord, I'm shy to present.

Through this poem, Tao tactfully declined the emperor's invitation, expressing his joy in a simple life and his wish to remain detached from worldly affairs. Tao Hongjing devoted himself to in-depth study of Daoism. He further developed the Supreme Clarity (*Shang Qing Dao*) and became the real founder of Mao Shan (Mt. Mao) Sect. He has been considered as an eminent and influential Daoist figure in the Southern dynasty (420–589). His book *Records on Nourishing Character & Prolonging Life* (*Yang Xing Yan Ming Lu*) summarized the principles and practice on nurturing life before the Wei and Jin period (220–420). Some movements recorded in this book (e.g., draw a blow to left and right, hold up the heaven using alternate hands, and two hands hold the feet, etc.) are very similar to *Ba Duan Jin* movements (e.g., look back to alleviate overstrain and emotions; bounce seven times on the feet, toes, heel; draw the bow to shoot the hawk; raise hand on each side to adjust the spleen & stomach, and clench the fists and glare fiercely to increase general vitality and muscular strength, etc.) in the late Qing dynasty (1644–1911).

The term of *Ba Duan Jin* was first recorded as *Longevity and Wellness Exercise* (*Chang Sheng An Le Fa*) in the *Yi Jian Zhi* by Hong Mai in the Song dynasty (960–1279); however, there were no detailed movements in the book. The *Jun Zhai Du Shu Zhi* compiled by Chao Gongwu in 1151 states, "*Ba Duan Jin* (whose author is unknown) is about rhymes of breathing out the stale and breathing in the fresh." Unfortunately this book was lost. Lu You[1] (1125–1210) mentioned in the *Qing Zun Lu* that General Yao Pingzhong in Northern Song dynasty (960–1126) had taught *Ba Duan Jin* in Mount Lu.

Zeng Zao, an eminent Daoist scholar in early years of the Southern Song dynasty recorded *Ba Duan Jin* in annotations of the 23rd volume (*Lin Jiang Xian*, literally means Immortals on the River) of the *Xiu Zhen Shi Shu Za Zhu Jie Jing* (*Shortcut to Miscellaneous Writings, Ten Books on Cultivating Perfection*). According to the original text, Lü Dongbin[2] carved the *Ba Duan Jin* of Zhongli Quan[3] on the stone wall to pass down through generations. Thereafter, *Ba Duan Jin* of Dou Yinqing and Mr. Cui had been supplemented (unfortunately, these two versions were lost). Zeng Zao supplemented six-word healing sounds. The verses and interpretations of Zeng Zao *Ba Duan Jin* and Zhongli *Ba Duan Jin* are as follows:

Zeng Zao *Ba Duan Jin* (Volume 23, *Xiu Zhen Shi Shu Za Zhu Jie Jing*, Photocopy of Daozang, the Cultural Relics Publishing House, 1988):

Time: 11 pm–1 am; 3 am–4 am

Sit down with a concentrated mind. Click the teeth (36 times) and hear the heavenly drum (36 times). Lift the arms up (three times coupled with the healing sound of "*xi*"). Then flex the thumb under the other four fingers to press the thigh (three

---

1 Lu You: a prominent poet of China's Southern Song dynasty (1127–1276).

2 Lü Dongbin: One of the earliest masters of Neidan or internal alchemy, a Tang dynasty scholar and poet who has been elevated to the status of an Immortal in the Chinese cultural sphere.

3 Zhongli Quan: Courtesy name Yun Fang, one of the most ancient of the Eight Immortals and the leader of the group. He is also known as Zhongli of Han because he was said to be born during the Han dynasty (202 BC–AD 220).

times on each side, right thigh first), coupled with the healing sound of "*xu*" for left side and the healing sound of "*dao*" for right side). Twist the hands and rub the eyes (seven times, close the eyes and turn the eyeballs seven times, and twist Taiyang, an extra acupuncture point 36 times using the knuckle of the middle finger), draw a bow (20 or 30 times on each side coupled with the healing sound of "*he*") and step the crossbow (three times on each side, three times of drawing the bow and seven times of stepping the crossbow, coupled with the healing sound of "*he*"), and rotate the body like a pulley (rotate the body 36 times on each side coupled with the healing sound of "*chui*").

Conduct three times of *Chao Yuan*[1] (pressing the legs, closing the eyes and swallowing *qi* coupled with the healing sound of "*chui*"), followed by nine times of imagining that *qi* from the Dantian moving. After this, sit with crossed feet, hold the breath, twist the hands until they become warm and rub the surrounding area of Shenshu acupoint (BL 23)[2], coupled with the healing sound of "*chui*." Then press the legs, close the eyes, hold the breath and rotate the body to each side for a couple of times, coupled with the healing sound of "*he*." Pull the feet with the hands coupled with the healing sound of "*he*" and grasp the heels (three times for each foot) coupled with the healing sound of "*hu*." Touch the upper palate using the tongue to produce saliva, rinse the mouth 36 times with the saliva, swallow in three gulps and imagine descending the saliva to the Dantian. Repeat three times coupled with the healing sound of "*chui*." Breathe in through the

1 A health cultivation practice in Daoism to gather *qi* of five-*zang* organs into the umbilicus.

2 Shenshu (BL 23): An acupuncture point located in the depression below the spinous process of the 2nd lumbar vertebra, 1.5 cun lateral to the posterior midline.

nose, hold the breath, twist the hands until they become warm and then rub the body until presence of mild sweats. Raise left and right arms to ascend *qi* sensation to ten fingernails. Finally, pronounce the healing sounds of "*chui*" (for the kidney), "*he*" (for the heart), "*xu*" (for the liver), "*xi*" (for *Sanjiao*), "*dao*" (for the lung) and "*hu*" (for the spleen) silently.

Zhongli *Ba Duan Jin* (Volume 19, *Xiu Zhen Shi Shu Za Zhu Jie Jing*):

Sit down with eyes closed and mind concentrated (concentrate the mind and sit with legs crossed). Flex the thumb under the other four fingers and click teeth 36 times. Cross the fingers, place them over the occiput and count nine times of breaths silently (Do not make it audible. After that, keep the inhalation and exhalation inaudible).

Then, sound the left and right heavenly drums for 24 times (cover both ears with the centers of palms. First press the middle finger with the index finger and then tap the occiput 24 times on each side using the index finger).

Slightly sway to shake the heavenly pillar (Turn the head to the left and right, eyes looking backwards as far as possible. Move the shoulders and arms simultaneously. Repeat 24 times on each side. Be sure to flex the thumb under the other four fingers first).

The red dragon stirs the water (The red dragon here refers to the tongue. Touch the teeth, gum and upper palate using the tip of the tongue to produce saliva). Rinse the mouth with the saliva 36 times (also known as drum rinsing) until your mouth becomes filled with saliva, swallow it in three gulps with a gurgling sound. In this way, the dragon (fluid) and tiger (*qi*) will naturally run (circulate smoothly).

Hold the breath and rub the hands until they become warm (Take a deep breath through the nose and hold it for a while.

Rub the hands until they become really warm. Then slowly breathe out). Then use the palms to rub the *Jingmen* on the back (*Jingmen* literally means essential gate, here refers to the kidney). Return and flex the thumb under the other four fingers. After this breath is exhausted (hold the breath again), imagine fire burning the Manipura (hold the breath in the mouth and nose and imagine sending heart fire down to burn the Dantian area until you feel extremely warm).

Rotate the body to the left and right like a pulley (lower the head and shake shoulders 36 times to each side. Imaging the fire from Dantian to ascend through the Jia Ji pass[1] and Yu Zhen pass[2] and enter the brain. Take a deep breath through the nose and hold it for a while). Relax both legs (stretch both legs).

Cross hands and raise the palms up (cross both hands and push them up for three or nine times).

Lower the head and touch the feet with both hands (Touch the soles using both hands 12 times. Then return the feet and sit upright). Wait for the water to ascend (Wait for the saliva to be produced in the mouth. If it does not appear, use the aforementioned method to produce saliva). Then rinse the mouth and swallow the saliva. Repeat this three times and swallow the divine water (saliva) nine times (this means to rinse the mouth for 36 times more and then swallow it in three gulps as mentioned above). Swallow with a gurgling sound. This can harmonize all channels.

---

1 One the of the three passes, also known as the Lu Lu pass or double Jia Ji passes. Location: on the back and at the midpoint of the line connecting bilateral olecranon in a prone position.

2 One of the three passes in the occiput, Yu Zhen literally means the Jade Pillow. Location: slightly below the point Yuzhen (BL 9) and in between bilateral Fengchi (GB 20). It is the last pass along the Governor Vessel that the internal *qi* has to overcome.

Along with a smooth circulation of *qi* and blood within the microcosmic and macrocosmic orbits, (sway the shoulders and the body 24 times coupled with 24 times of rotating the body like a pulley), start the fire to burn the entire body (imagine that Dantian fire burns the entire body from bottom to top. At the same time, hold the breath in the mouth and nose for a while). This will keep away evil spirits and pathogenic factors and result in good sleep. This exercise should be done after the period between 11 pm and 1 am and before the period between 11 pm and 1 am. It's advisable to follow the sequence of the eight movements and directions.

The verses states, "... during *Ba Duan Jin* exercise, breathe through the nose instead of the mouth. This exercise can be practiced two or three times a day. Over time, this can help remove chronic conditions and promote health. Perseverant exercise can even help one achieve longevity."

Zhongli *Ba Duan Jin* contains verses and illustrations. As for verses, they are 36 five-word rhymes coupled with annotations. As for movements in a sitting position, these include mental focus combined with clicking the teeth, swallowing the saliva, rubbing the back and low back, rotating the shoulder, extending the leg, reaching to grasp the feet with hands, etc. Originally there are eight illustrations; however, there are no names recorded for these illustrations.

In the 35th volume (*Zhong Miao Pian,* the *Chapter of Wonders*) of *Dao Shu* (*The Pivot of Dao*) by Zeng Zao, seven movements were recorded as follows: Lift arms and turn palms to the sky to regulate *Sanjiao*, draw a bow to both sides to shoot a hawk, left for the liver and right for the lung, raise one hand up east and west to harmonize the spleen and stomach, look back and forward to regulate emotions, gather *qi* of five-*zang* organs to Dantian area, swallow saliva to supplement *qi*, flick all fingers and sweep the tail like an eel to remove heart problems and reach the feet with both hands to strengthen the low back.

In the *Xiu Zhen Mi Zhi*, *Shi Lin Guang Ji* (*The Secret of Health, the Encyclopedia*) by Cheng Yuanjing in the Southern Song dynasty, *Lü Zhenren* (i.e., Lü Dongbin) *An Li Fa* was recorded as follows: Raise the head and lift palms to the sky to regulate *Sanjiao*, draw a bow to both sides to shoot a hawk, left for the liver and right for the lung, lift hand to the east to regulate the spleen and to the west to regulate the stomach, look back and forward to balance seven emotions, sweep the tail like an eel to benefit heart *qi*, reach the feet with both hands to strengthen the low back, gather *qi* of five-*zang* organs to Dantian area and swallow saliva and flick fingers on both hands.

Although these descriptions did not mention the name of *Ba Duan Jin*, they are very similar to the later verses of *Ba Duan Jin* and therefore considered as its prototypes.

The early versions of *Ba Duan Jin* include practice in a standing/sitting position, *Dao Yin* alone, six healing sounds coupled with *Dao Yin* or *Dao Yin* coupled with *Tu Na* (inhalation and exhalation), etc.

The well-known *Ba Duan Jin Dao Yin* method was recorded in *Huo Ren Xin Fa* (*The Method of Saving People*) by Zhu Quan (1378–1448), the 17th son of Zhu Yuanzhang (Ming Taizu, 1328–1398, the founder and first emperor of the Ming dynasty). Today, this set of exercises can still be found in the Korean woodblock-printed editions such as *Bao Sheng Xin Jian* (*Personal Experience in Health Cultivation*) (1506) attached to the *Huo Ren Xin Fa* and a North Korean book *Yi Fang Lei Ju* (*Categorized Collection of Medical Formulas*). With a perfect combination of motion (active exercises) and stillness (tranquil inner cultivation), *Ba Duan Jin Dao Yin* has played an important role in the history of Chinese *Yangsheng* (life-nurturing) and *Dao Yin*.

Later, the "Zhongli (sitting) *Ba Duan Jin*" was referenced in many medical and health cultivation books in the Ming (1368–1644) and Qing dynasties, including *Lei Xiu Yao Jue* (*The Essence of Categorized Exercises*) (1592), *Zun Sheng Ba Jian,Yan Nian Que Bing Jian* (*Achieving Longevity and Removing Diseases, Health Cultivation in Eight Ways*) (1591), *Yi Men Guang Du*, *Chi Feng Sui* (*Marrow of Red Phoenix, Archives By a Hermit*) (1579), *Xiu Ling Yao Zhi* (*The Essence of Health Cultivation Exercise*) (approximately 1642). *She Sheng Zong Yao* (*General Principle for Health Cultivation*) (1638), *Wan Shou Xian Shu* (*Treatises on Longevity and Immortality*) (1632) and *San Cai Tu Hui* (*Assembled Illustrations of Heaven, Earth and Man*).

Books in the Qing dynasty and North Korean documents frequently featured *Ba Duan Jin* verses and illustrations of *Ba Duan Jin* in sitting positions, marking a flourishing period for *Dao Yin* practices during the Ming and Qing dynasties.

Historically, there are other recordings of *Ba Duan Jin* verses. The *Lei Xiu Yao Jue* (*The Essence of Categorized Exercises*) in the Ming dynasty cited *Ling Jian Zi Yin Dao Zi Wu Ji*, *Yin Dao Jue* and renamed it *Xu Zhen Jun Yin Dao Jue*. The *Yi Fang Lei Ju* (*Categorized Collection of Medical Formulas*) by Jin Limeng from Korea recorded *Lü Zhen Ren* (i.e., Lü Dongbin) *An Le Fa*. The *Yi Yang Quan Yao* (*Elaboration Summary of Health Conservation*) by Feng Xi in the Qing dynasty recorded similar *Lü Zu* (i.e., *Lü Dongbin) An Le Ge*. After studying *Ba Duan Jin* in both standing and sitting positions, Lou Jie in the Qing dynasty compiled the *Ba Duan Jin Zuo Li Gong Fa Tu Jue* (*Illustrated Ba Duan Jin Verses in Standing and Sitting Positions*) in 1876 (the 2nd year of Guangxu era). Today, *Fang Cao Xuan* woodblock-printed edition (1876) of this book is still available, coupled with the Guangzhou Shou Jing Tang woodblock-printed edition of *Ba Duan Jin Tu Shuo* (*Illustrated Ba Duan Jin*) by Qing Lai Zhen Ren in the Qing dynasty.

According to the textual research by Tang Hao[1], most popular dynamic *Ba Duan Jin* movements and verses were formed in the Guangxu period (1875–1908). The *You Xue Cao Shen* (*Physical Exercises for Children*) published by Shanghai Tongwen Shuju[2] in 1890 and the *Xin Chu Bao Shen Tu, Ba Duan Jin Tu* (*Ba Duan Jin Movements in Illustrated New Methods for Health Preservation*) published in 1898 recorded the following seven-character verse:

Lifting the heavens with two hands to regulate Sanjiao
Drawing the bow both left and right-handed to shoot the hawk
Holding one arm aloft to regulate the spleen and stomach
Looking from side to side to prevent five overstrains and seven injuries[3]
Swaying the head and shaking to clear heart-fire
Seven times of bouncing to relieve all diseases
Clenching the fists and glaring angrily to increase strength
Holding the feet with both hands to consolidate the kidney and low back

Compared with the verses in the Ming and Qing dynasties, this verse is easier to learn and has become the most influential one, since it removed breathing in, breathing out and mental

---

1 Tang Hao (1887–1959): a Chinese lawyer and expert on Chinese martial arts. He published a dozen books on the history of Chinese martial arts.

2 Tongwen Shuju: the first lithographic printing house in the history of China, founded by Xu Xun and Xu Hongfu in 1882. Unfortunately, it was closed in 1898.

3 Five overstrains refer to damages to the liver, heart, spleen, lung and kidney; they may also refer to five causes of overstrains: long-time use of your eyes damages your blood, long-time sitting damages your muscles, long-term standing damages your bones, longtime walking damages your tendons and long-time bed rest damages your *qi*. Seven injuries refer to negative effects caused by extreme emotions such as joy, anger, worry, grief, sadness, fear and fright.

focus on Dantian and highlighted physical movements on the basis of *Ling Jian Zi Yin Dao Zi Wu Ji*, *Yin Dao Jue*. Later, *Ba Duan Jin* in sitting and standing positions are named Sitting *Ba Duan Jin* and Standing *Ba Duan Jin*. Further to this classification, standing *Ba Duan Jin* is subdivided into the Northern school and Southern school. The northern school, also known as the hard style, involves horse riding stance and tough movements; while the southern school, also known as the soft style, involves standing posture and gentle movements.

The *Ba Duan Jin* published by the People's Sports Publishing House of China in 1957 described the functions and practice tips of *Ba Duan Jin* and illustrated three sets of standing *Ba Duan Jin* by Zhuo Dahong, Ma Fengge and Tang Hao and one set of sitting *Ba Duan Jin* by Ma Fengge. With a huge number of printed copies, this easy-to-understand book has greatly contributed to the popularization and promotion of *Ba Duan Jin*.

In addition, there is also the Shaolin *Ba Duan Jin*. Some scholars believe *Ba Duan Jin* originated from Shaolin[1] *Yi Jin Jing* (*Sinew Transforming Classic*). As the old legend goes, Bodhidharma (from India) arrived in Guangzhou by sea in the era of Emperor Wu of the Southern Liang dynasty. After a brief and unsuccessful meeting with the emperor in Jianye (today's Nanjing in Jiangsu Province in eastern China), Bodhidharma was said to have crossed the river on a single stem of reed, travelled north to Luoyang, the capital of the Northern Wei dynasty (386–534) and settled at the Shaolin Temple on Mount Song, where he sat facing a wall without a word for nine years and finally created

1 Shaolin often refers to the Shaolin Monastery, or Shaolin Temple, a Buddhist monastery in Henan Province, China. Specifically, it refers to Shaolin Kung Fu, the school of martial arts associated with the monastery.

the *Yi Jin Jing*. Since *Yi Jin Jing* is difficult to learn, the Shaolin monks selected eight movements and named these movements *Ba Duan Jin*.

Ba Duan Jin was clearly explained in detail in the *Yi Jin Jing Wai Jing Tu Shuo*, *Wai Zhuang Lian Li Qi Yan Tu* (*Amazing Experience in Building Physical Strength, Illustrations of Yi Jin Jing Branches*) (unknown author in Qing dynasty) and *Ba Duan Jin Ti Cao Tu* (*Gymnastic Illustrations of 12 Ba Duan Jin Movements*). Along with the evolution of Shaolin Kung Fu (martial arts), Shaolin monks created their special Shaolin *Ba Duan Jin* by integrating *Ba Duan Jin*, Shaolin meditation and Shaolin martial arts with Chinese medical theories on *yin*, *yang*, five elements, internal organs and meridians & points. Buddhist monks practice Shaolin *Ba Duan Jin* as part of their daily training to preserve health, improve their martial arts skills and recover from injuries.

Some scholars believe *Ba Duan Jin* is another name of *Ba Duan Jin* (literally means Extreme Stretching of the Sinew) or *Qian Ba Zan Chu Ji Dao Gong* (Disease-Removing Daoist Exercise by Repeating 1,800 Times, indicating that it takes lots of practice to obtain remarkable effects), an active physical exercise in combination with tranquil inner cultivation. Daoist sages practiced this to stretch and transform sinew to compensate for the *qi* stagnation and blood exhaustion due to long-term sitting meditation. This exercise method was quoted in the *Wu Shu Hui Zong* (*Collections of Martial Arts*) by Wan Laisheng, a prominent 20th-century martial artist who learned from Wang Xianzhai, a hermit at the Baiyun (White Cloud) Daoist Temple in Beijing. Based on the Daoist theory of "harmony between man and nature," this exercise uses the body as a smaller heavenly cycle (microcosmic orbit), coincides with astrology of the world and universe and adopts movements corresponding to sun, moon, green dragon, white tiger, vermillion bird and black tortoise.

These profound movements are simple, gentle, smooth and continuous. Characterized by arm circling the front, back, left, right, upper part and lower part of the body, coupled with head rotation and rhythmic mild flexion and extension of the leg, this exercise can alleviate frozen shoulder and pain in the neck, low back and leg in middle-aged and elderly people. In addition, the word "*Zan*" (in *Qian Ba Zan Chu Ji Dao Gong*) means clenching a fist in each movement, which can benefit the heart and lung. Gentle smooth and continuous movements allow free flow of *qi* and blood in meridians. As a result, regular practice of these simple movements can promote health.

Based on essence (*Jing*), *qi* and spirit (*Shen*) as well as the theory "when there is sufficient healthy *qi* inside, the pathogenic *qi* have no way to invade the body" and "genuine *qi* will be with you when you achieve *Tian* (peaceful joy), *Dan* (no greed for fame and wealth), *Xu* (void) and *Wu* (nothingness)" in the *Huang Di Nei Jing* (*The Inner Canon of the Yellow Emperor*), the author revised through decades of practice and clinical studies. He especially attached much importance to one's character, quality and temperament. As for specific body movements, mental intention comes first. Consequently the revised *Ba Duan Jin* can help to nurture one's character, remove diseases and achieve health and longevity.

Theoretical Foundation

In terms of functions of body movements alone, *Ba Duan Jin* is similar to broadcast gymnastics and self-care massage. However, mental intention and essential *qi* are crucial to its function in nurturing one's character and promoting health. To fully understand spirit, essence, character and *qi*, one needs first to be familiar with basic concepts in traditional culture. In other words, one needs to understand the underlying truth before practice *Ba Duan Jin*. Otherwise, it's like "a blind man riding a blind horse approaches the brink of an unfathomable pool at midnight."

The Way to Pursue Underlying Truth

The theoretical system of the Chinese traditional culture is totally different from that of modern science. Modern science aims to pursue truth or knowledge of phenomena of the "physical world" and therefore highlights "physical evidence"; whereas the Chinese traditional culture focuses on "*Dao*"—the underlying natural order of the universe. The phenomena of the "physical world" are just the manifestation of "*Dao*"—a "phase" that changes all the time.

Dao can be thought of as the flow of the universe. The basic law of *Dao* is to transform from nothingness to existence. The *Dao De Jing*[1] states, "There was something undefined and complete, coming into existence before Heaven and Earth. We look at it, and we do not see it. We listen to it, and we do not hear it. How still it was and formless, standing alone, and undergoing no change, reaching everywhere and in no danger of being exhausted! It may be regarded as the Mother of all things. I do not know its name, and I give it the designation of the *Dao*." This text says, "Conceived of as having no name, it is the Originator of heaven and earth; conceived of as having a name, it is the Mother of all things," and "the *Dao* produced One; One produced Two; Two produced Three; Three produced All Things." The law of the *Dao* is its being what it is.

Chapter 66 of the *Huang Di Nei Jing Su Wen* states, "the extension of the Great Void is boundless; it is the basis of all

1 Also simply referred to as the *Laozi*, is a Chinese classic text. According to tradition, it was written around 6th century BC by the sage Laozi.

founding and it is the principal source of all transformation. The myriad beings depend on the Great Void to come into existence, and it is because of the Great Void that the five movements (*Wu Yun*) complete their course in heaven. The Great Void spreads the true magic power of *qi*, and it exerts control over the principal *qi* of the earth. Hence the nine stars are suspended in heaven and shine and the seven luminaries revolve in a cycle. This is called *yin*; this is called *yang*. This is called soft; this is called hard. Hence when that which is in the dark and that which is obvious have assumed their positions, there is cold and summer-heat, tension and relaxation. Generation follows upon generation, transformation follows upon transformation, with the result that all the things come into open existence."

From the perspective of traditional Daoist culture, the above theoretical system can be summarized into *Dao* (natural order) → *qi* (transformation) → physical world (changes). Unlike modern scientific view, Daoism believes there are changes of *qi* and *Dao* before the material world. The *Yi Men Fa Lü* (*Precepts for Medical Practice*) (1658) says, "When *qi* gathers, the physical body is formed; when *qi* disperses, the body dies." This can be best explained from the following story *Zhuang Zi's Wife Died*.

When Zhuangzi's wife died, Hui Shi came to condole. As for Zhuangzi, he was squatting with his knees out, drumming on a pot and singing. "When you have lived with someone," said Hui Shi, "and brought up children, and grown old together, to refuse to bewail her death would be bad enough, but to drum on a pot and sing—could there be anything more shameful?" "Not so. When she first died, do you suppose that I was able not to feel the loss? I peered back into her beginnings; there was a time before there was a life. Not only was there no life, there was a time before there was a shape. Not only was there no shape, there was a time before there was energy. Mingled together in the amorphous, something altered, and there was the energy; by the alteration in the energy there was the shape, by alteration of the shape there was the life. Now once more altered, she has gone over to death. This is to be companion with spring and autumn, summer and winter, in the procession of the four seasons. When someone was about to lie down and sleep in the greatest of mansions, I with my sobbing knew no better than to bewail her. The thought came to me that I was being uncomprehending towards destiny, so I stopped weeping."

Apparently, *Dao* is the most fundamental element in the above theoretical system; and *qi* (transformation) and physical world (changes) are different forms of *Dao*. Therefore, it is important to comprehend and follow the *Dao*. Otherwise, it's like "going south by driving the chariot north (doing something counterproductive to one's goal)" to study "*Dao*" and "Logic" in traditional culture from the mindset of "physical evidence."

In essence, traditional health cultivation practice including *Ba Duan Jin* tends to return to the origin: physical world (changes) → *qi* (transformation) → *Dao* (natural order). They stress more on "cleansing and plifting" process, which paves the way for the cultivation of essence, *qi* and spirit or temperament, and for exploring the deep interplay between the mind and *qi*.

The Origin of *Zhen* (Genuine) *Qi*

Qigong practice pursues *Zhen* (genuine) *qi* and *Zheng* (healthy/positive) *qi*, which are closely associated with "*Dao*" and "*De*" (virtue).

Dao is the underlying natural order of the universe. The *Zhou Yi*[1] *Xi Ci* (*Philosophical Interpretation on the Book of Changes*) states, "One *Yin* and One *Yang* are called *Dao*" and "the *Dao* of heaven

1 An ancient divination text and the oldest of the Chinese classics.

is known as *yin* and *yang*." Confucius believed "what is above the form (metaphysical) is called *Dao*; what is under the form (physical) is called a tool." As a result, "*Dao* is the interaction between *yin* and *yang*."

De (virtue) is the inherent nature or character. The *Mengzi* (*Mencius*) states, "the feeling of commiseration is essential to man, that the feeling of shame and dislike is essential to man, that the feeling of modesty and complaisance is essential to man, and that the feeling of approving and disapproving is essential to man. The feeling of commiseration is the principle of benevolence. The feeling of shame and dislike is the principle of righteousness. The feeling of modesty and complaisance is the principle of propriety. The feeling of approving and disapproving is the principle of knowledge. Men have these four principles just as they have their four limbs. Yet, they just do not realize they have them."

Dao and *De* were first used in combination in the "Quan Xue" (the chapter of "Persuading/Encouraging Learning") by Xun Zi[1] as "... therefore learning reaches its completion with the rituals, for they may be said to represent the highest point of *Dao De* (inner strength/personal character)." Today, "*Dao De*" is a social ideology, referring to a body of standards or principles derived from a code of conduct. It can be seen that the word "*Dao De*" in traditional culture is far more profound than in modern text.

Basic Concept of *Qi*

Qi is the most essential substance that constitutes the universe and human body and acts to maintain vital activities. It can be

---

1 Along with Confucius and Mencius, Xun Zi was one of the three great early architects of Confucian philosophy.

understood from energy and functions.

Energy. Energy here includes clean *qi*, nutrients *qi* from water and grains and *yuan*-primordial *qi*. An example can help us understand clean *qi*. After living in a city for a long period of time, we feel refreshed when we travel to a place with fresh air, because we breathed in fresh air from the nature through our lung. As for nutrients *qi*, we need energy from water and food through our stomach and intestines. *Yuan*-primordial *qi* is inherited from one's parents, just like some kids are born weak, some strong, some smart and some relatively dull.

Functions. Functions of *qi* include *qi* activity, vital activity, mental intention and regulation. For example, anger causes *qi* to ascend, leading to a red face and elevated blood pressure.

However, the aforementioned *qi* is not the "*qi*" we pursued in *qigong* practice. As we mentioned before, *qigong* practice pursues *Zhen* (genuine) *qi* and *Zheng* (healthy/positive) *qi* that are closely associated with "*Dao*" and "*De* (virtue)." This is what we say "when there is sufficient healthy *qi* inside, the pathogenic *qi* have no way to invade the body" and "genuine *qi* will be with you when you achieve *Tian* (peaceful joy), *Dan* (no greed for fame and wealth), *Xu* (void) and *Wu* (nothingness)." To acquire *Zhen qi* and *Zheng qi*, we need to follow *Dao* and cultivate our virtue. The *Dao De Jing* states, "All things are produced by the *Dao*, and nourished by the *De* (virtue). They receive their forms according to the nature of each, and are completed according to the circumstances of their condition. Therefore all things without exception honor the *Dao*, and exalt the virtue. This honoring of the *Dao* and exalting of its operation is not the result of any ordination, but always a spontaneous tribute." In summary, "*Dao*" produces all things and "*De*" nourishes all things. The outer chapter *Heaven and Earth* in *Zhuangzi* states, "pervading heaven and earth, that is the *Dao*; moving among the ten thousand things, that is the *De*." This chapter also states, "Without *Dao*, the body can have no life. Without *De*, life can have no clarity. To preserve the body and live out life, to establish *De* and clarify *Dao*—is this not kingly (*De*) virtue?" Mencius says, "I'm good at nourishing my flood-like righteous *qi* ..." He goes on to describe what means by "flood-like righteous *qi*": It is the sort of *qi* utmost in vastness and power. If, by uprightness, you nourish it and do not interfere with it, it fills the space between Heaven and Earth. It is the sort of *qi* that matches virtue and morality; without these, it starves. It is generated by the accumulation of virtue and morality—one cannot attain it by sporadic righteousness. If anything one does fail to meet the standards of one's heart-mind, it starves.

The principle of our revised *Ba Duan Jin* lies in the "genuine *qi* will be with you when you achieve *Tian* (peaceful joy), *Dan* (no greed for fame and wealth), *Xu* (void) and *Wu* (nothingness)." *Tian*, *Dan*, *Xu* and *Wu* are four levels of following the *Dao*. *Tian* means tranquil, serene and joyful. This peaceful joy arises from the inner heart and has nothing to do with gain and loss in real life. *Dan* means not to seek fame and wealth. One can only determine his/her aspiration by not seeking secular fame and wealth; one can only achieve his/her ambition by having a tranquil peaceful mind. *Xu* and *Wu* are more difficult to explain. These four levels can be explained from the following example (metaphor). Imagine you are in a room with a closed door, windows and thick wool curtain. You cannot see your own fingers in this dark room. This is a normal state of ordinary people. When the curtain is pulled aside, the sunlight enters the room, allowing you to see the scene outside through the window. This is the first level "*Tian*." When the door and windows are open, you feel the room is connected with the outside world. This is the second level of "*Dan*." When you are still in the room but feel like the house is absent, this is the third level of "*Xu*" When you forget yourself, this is the fourth level of "*Wu*."

During *qigong* practice, to connect with the *Zhen* (genuine) *qi* between the heaven and earth, you need to forget yourself in tranquil stillness. This can be vividly reflected in a poem by Zhu Xi[1]:

A small square pond an uncovered mirror,
Where sunlight and clouds linger and leave.
I asked how it stays so clear,
It said spring water keeps flowing in.

Through *qigong* practice, we can seek the truth about our life and universe. Through *qigong* practice, we are willing to assume responsibility of our life. The *Yi Jing* (*Book of Changes*) states, "As Heaven keeps vigor through movement, a gentleman should unremittingly practice self-improvement. As the earth bears everything on it, a gentleman should generously cultivate to become tolerant."

Differences Between *Ba Duan Jin* Practice and Modern Physical Exercise

Unlike modern sports training, traditional *qigong* practices reflect deep cultural roots and emphasize individualized cultivation. Their uniqueness lies in their teaching principles, movement requirements, and underlying theoretical system.

Difference in teaching method. Student-tailored teaching methods are often adopted in traditional *qigong* learning.

1 A Song dynasty Confucian scholar who became the leading figure of the School of Principle and the most influential rationalist Neo-Confucian in China.

Considering from individualized constitution and lifestyles, even for same exercise, some can begin with static meditation, some with active body movements, some with "essence," some with "*qi*" and some with "spirit." Due to diffcrences in gift and knowledge in traditional culture, some can begin with the whole (*Dao*), some with a part, some with inaction, some with action, some with mental intention and some with body movements.

Above all, teachers play the most important role in learning traditional *qigong* exercise. Experience, guidance and instruction of teachers are extremely significant.

Difference in key principles and movement requirements. Under the framework of scientific theory, movements are unified and standardized. However, traditional health cultivation practice varies greatly between different schools. Movements may also vary among students even though they learn from the same teacher, since traditional *qigong* practice focuses more on mental intention than specific movements. Due to differences in understanding the underlying idea, gender and age, there are appropriate movements instead of fixed, standardized ones.

Difference in theoretical system. Modern physical exercise, body building exercise and recuperative gymnastics are based on human anatomy, physiology and biochemical indices.

Based on *Dao* (natural order) → *qi* (transformation) → physical world (changes), *yin-yang* changes, five-*zang* organs, circulation of *qi* and blood along meridians, traditional health cultivation practice aims to achieve moderation and balance through exercise in the right place at the right time.

Chapter Two
Characteristics and Essential Principles

Traditional health cultivation is not merely about physical exercise—it is a holistic practice of uniting body and mind, a journey of returning to one's true nature. The following points reveal its unique training principles and profound spiritual essence.

Living a Vigorous Life

It's generally believed that *Yang Sheng* (Nurturing Life) means physical fitness. However, in addition to physical body, Chinese medicine highlights body-mind balance. When we say nurturing life, we mean the most original vigor of life—vital *qi*. Physical body is just a concrete manifestation of vital *qi*. What is the origin of "vital *qi*?" Chapter 74 of the *Huang Di Nei Jing* states, "seasonal changes of the nature correspond with changes inside the human body." Chapter 66 of the *Huang Di Nei Jing* states, "In heaven it is *qi*; on the earth it turns into physical appearance. Physical appearance and *qi* affect each other and thereby they generate, through transformation, the myriad beings." As a result, the vital *qi* originates from *Dao*. In nature, *Dao* and man are one. If things are looked at in an isolated, partial and obsessive way, man and *Dao* will be separated into two. This can be explained from a glass of water and the ocean. In nature, a glass of water and the ocean are both water. The glass of water will evaporate if it's separated from the ocean. When the glass of water is poured into the sea, they become one. *Dao* of the heaven is to vital *qi* what the ocean is to the glass of water. If we understand *Dao*, we know "the glass of water is the ocean"; if we are with the *Dao*, we know "the ocean is the glass of water." In traditional culture, sages and men with great virtue believed "Life is a dream walking; death is a going home" and "Death is just a part of the life circulation, so the death is the birth."

We conduct life-nurturing practice not because we are scared of death and cravenly cling to life. Confucius once said, "if you don't know life, how can you know death?" Only by living a life, can we thoroughly understand and follow the *Dao* between heaven and earth. Zhang Zai (1020–1077)[1] is most known for laying out four ontological goals for intellectuals: to build up the manifestations of Heaven and Earth's spirit, to build up good life for the public, to develop past sages' endangered scholarship, and to open up eternal peace for generation after generation. With this spirit, one can live even after death. However, for those with "deep desires but shallow Heavenly sensitivities" (quotes from *Zhuangzi*), their lives are already death.

Intention Acts as the King, Whereas Bones/ Muscles Are Just Ministers

Xing means our body, including skin, muscle and internal organs, whereas *Shen* means our mind, including personality, willpower, emotions and mindset. Mind acts as the host and

1 A Chinese Neo-Confucian moral philosopher and cosmologist in the Song dynasty.

body as the house. In traditional *qigong* practice, intention acts as the king and bones/muscles are just ministers.

Stress in modern society can damage our health, causing depression, anxiety and physical imbalances. What's more, a huge volume of information, sensual pleasure and nightlife compromised our immune system. Chapter 12 of the *Dao De Jing* states, "The five colors blind the eye. The five tones deafen the ear. The five flavors dull the taste. Racing and hunting madden the mind. Precious things lead one astray. Therefore the sage is guided by what he feels and not by what he sees. He lets go of that and chooses this." Since one tends to be lost in excessive material desire, it's essential to pursue the natural vigor of life—vital *qi* in life nurturing exercise. The vital *qi* resides in the Dantian area. To activate vital *qi*, we need to guide our mental intent to the *Dao*. The genuine *qi* will be with us if we can achieve four levels of *Tian*, *Dan*, *Xu* and *Wu*. The "genuine *qi*," i.e., the "vital *qi*" can nourish internal organs, regulate meridians and help us stay healthy.

Combination of Stillness and Motion

As for stillness, the *Dao De Jing* states, "Empty you of everything. Let the mind become still. The ten thousand things rise and fall while the Self watches their return. They grow and flourish and then return to the source. Returning to the source is stillness, which is the way of nature."

As for motion, the *Lü Zu Bai Zi Ming* (*Hundred Words Stele by Lü Dongbin*) says, "the real ordinary mind should response to object sensed, but in responding should not get lost."

Active body movements need to be integrated into tranquil inner cultivation, just like the combination of *yin* softness and *yang* strength. According to the *Huang Di Nei Jing*, "long-time use of your eyes damages your blood, long-time sitting damages your muscles, long-term standing damages your bones, longtime walking damages your tendons and long-time bed rest damages your *qi*." Life can only be nurtured by balanced stillness and motion.

Keep Your Body and Mind Upright

The *Huang Di Nei Jing* states, "when there is sufficient healthy *qi* inside, the pathogenic *qi* have no way to invade the body." An upright mind leads to an upright body, which further leads to a smooth flow of *qi* and blood. When there is sufficient healthy *qi* in our body and mind, exogenous pathogens have no way to attack us. An upright body can help with concentration and free flow of *qi*. For beginners, it's extremely important to keep the body upright. Simply put, one needs to keep Baihui (GV 20)[1] and Huiyin (CV 1)[2] in the same line and stay comfortable. A good body posture can benefit *qi* activity. Regulating posture means to regulate internal organs, meridians, four limbs and essence, one of the Three Treasures—along with *qi* and spirit. Regulating the body means to regulate the relative movements and locations of sinew, fascia, bones and muscles. The priority of *qigong* practice is to focus on mind and *qi*, followed by body movements. In other words, it is important to use intent to guide posture and use *qi* to adjust posture.

1 An acupuncture point located at the intersection of the line connecting both ear tips and the midline of the head.

2 An acupuncture point located at the midpoint between the root of the scrotum and the anus in males, and at the midpoint between the female posterior labial commissure and the anus in females.

Chapter Three
Movements of *Ba Duan Jin*

This chapter begins with the two basic movements of *Ba Duan Jin*, highlighting their importance and laying a solid foundation for further study. It then provides a detailed analysis of the eight main movements of *Ba Duan Jin*, offering step-by-step demonstrations and key insights to help readers master the core skills and health benefits of *Ba Duan Jin* through systematic practice.

Basic Postures

Before learning the eight main movements of *Ba Duan Jin*, it is essential to first master two basic movements. Though simple in appearance, they form the foundation for subsequent movements and are vital for enhancing both exercise effectiveness and body coordination.

Stand in the *Wu Ji* Position

Description: Place your feet shoulder-width apart, slightly bend your knees (but do not let your knees extend past your toes), hang your arms loosely at your sides and keep your eyes half open and gaze down along the line of the nose.

Explanation: The essential concept of this posture is to "*Bao Yuan*." The first word "*Bao*" means to mix with or to embrace.

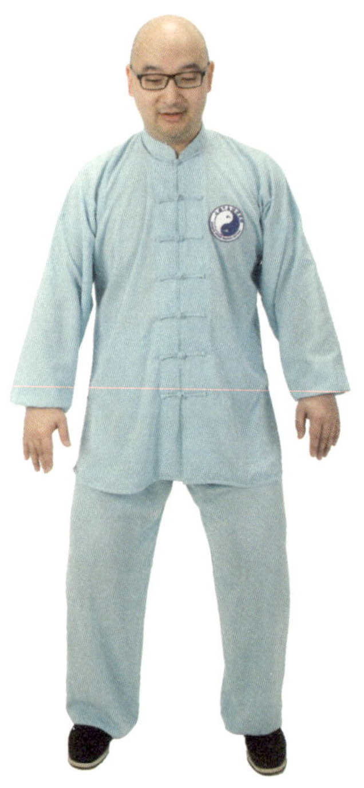

Fig. 1 Stand in the *Wu Ji* position.

The second word "*Yuan*" means *Wu Ji* (nothingness), the primordial origin, the root or the *Dao*. The "*Dao*" is the spontaneous way that all things began, the foundation of all intangible and invisible "substances" and activities, and the mother of all things in the universe. In summary, everything comes from the *Dao*. This standing posture requires a state of mindfulness, not-self and inaction, coupled with ascent of clean *yang* and descent of turbid *yin*.

Stand with Imagination of Holding a Ball

Description: Place your feet shoulder-width apart, slightly bend your knees and do not let your knees go past your toes, and then gently raise your arms until your hands are in front of your chest.

Explanation: The core of this posture is to "Embrace the One." "Embrace" here means never leave or give up. "The One" means *Taiji*, a state before separation of *yin* and *yang*. The *Dao De Jing* states, "there were those in old times who grasped and were possessed of the One: The heaven was much clarified by attaining it. Likewise, the earth got stable or calm by the same 'rotating' measure; and demon spirits or gods were spiritualized, and became divine. The valley likewise became full, the abyss replenished. By staying in the One, all creatures lived and grew." The *Tai Ping Jing*[1] (*Scripture of the Great Peace*) states, "the One is the guiding principle of heaven and origin of all things," and "the One is the root of *Dao* and beginning of *qi*." The *Zhuangzi* states, "that which is so great that there is nothing outside it can be called the Great One; and that which is so small that there is nothing inside it can be called the Small One."

Characteristics of this posture: Integrated motion and stillness and mutual dependence of mind and *qi*. Externally, it looks relaxed. Internally, the mind is cultivated. Use the vitality of innate *qi* to melt down turbid postnatal *qi*. Use mental intent to guide *qi* and *qi* always flows with the mind. In the end, you are with the nature and *Dao*.

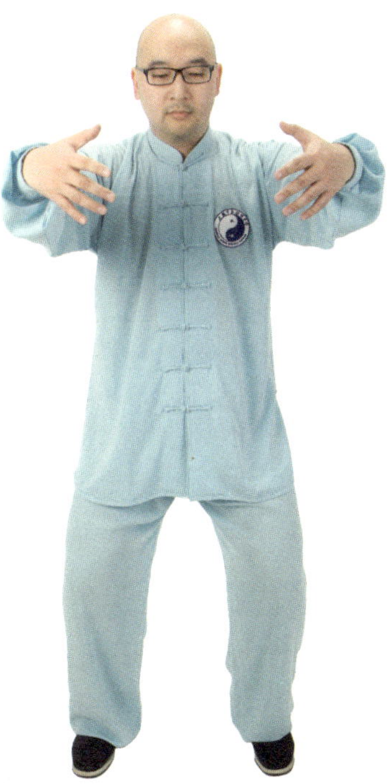

Fig. 2 Stand with imagination of holding a ball.

1 *Tai Ping Jing* often refers to the work which has been preserved in the *Daozang*. It is considered to be a valuable resource for researching early Daoist beliefs and the society at the end of the Eastern Han dynasty (25–220).

Individual Movements

Then, we will carefully analyze the steps and principles of the eight movements of *Ba Duan Jin* using both images and text.

Movement One: Lift the Heavens with Two Hands to Regulate *Sanjiao*

About this movement: This movement focuses on ascending and descending of *qi* in *Sanjiao*. It enables *qi* and *yang* to ascend and *yin* and blood to descend. Stretching of the four limbs and torso can regulate associated muscles, bones and ligaments and prevent or treat pain in the arms, neck, shoulder and low back.

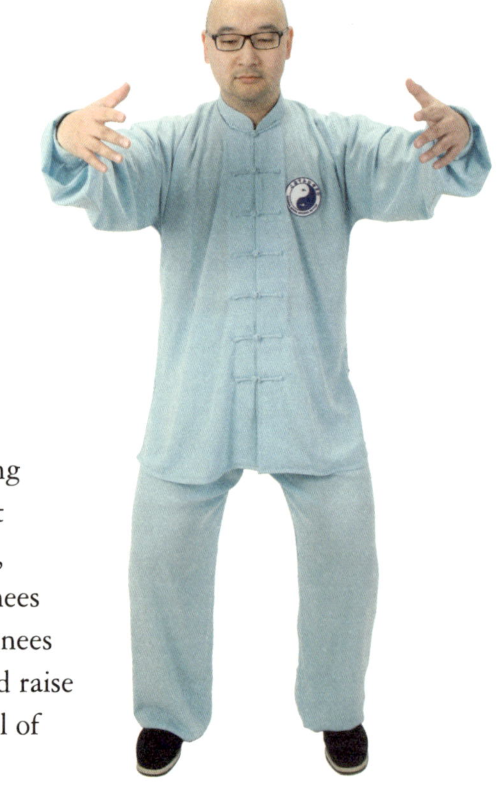

❶

1. Standing with imagination of holding a ball: Place your feet shoulder width apart, slightly bend your knees and do not let your knees go past your toes, and raise your arms to the level of your chest.

2. Slowly drop the hands along both sides of the body and put two hands together in front of the lower abdomen.

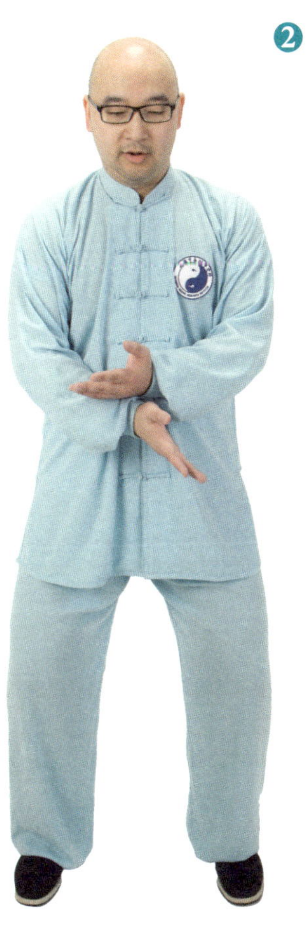

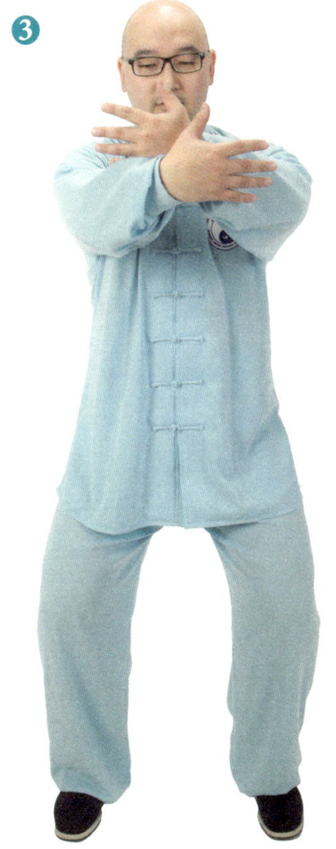

3. Lift the hands to the level of chest, slightly forward.

4. Turn the palms up and rise above the head.

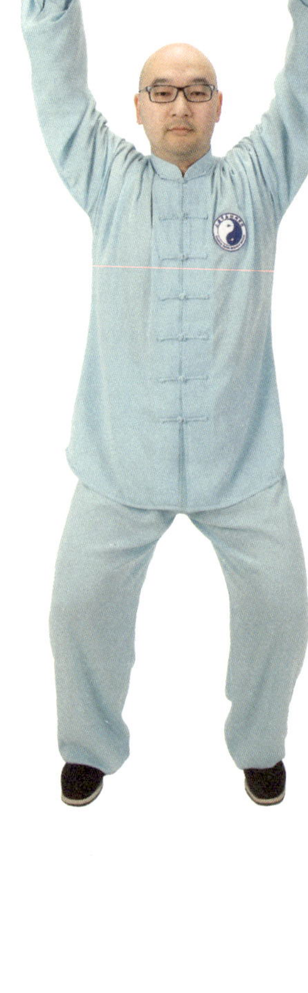

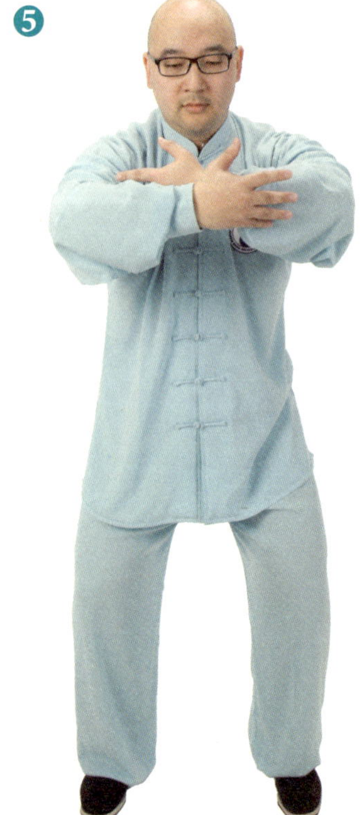

5. Open the hands from above the head to both side and close them in front of the chest.

6. Open the hands in front of the chest again.

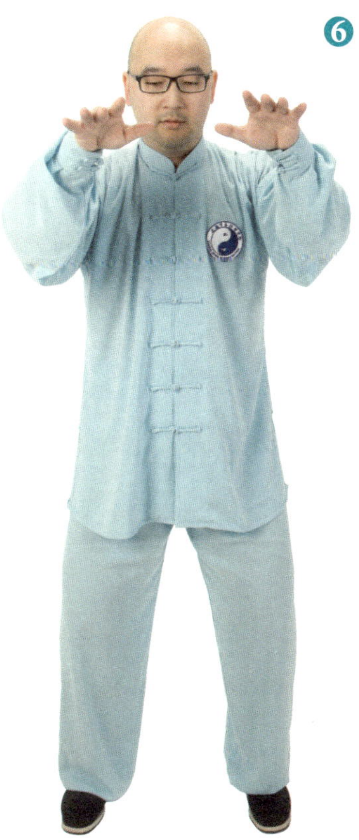

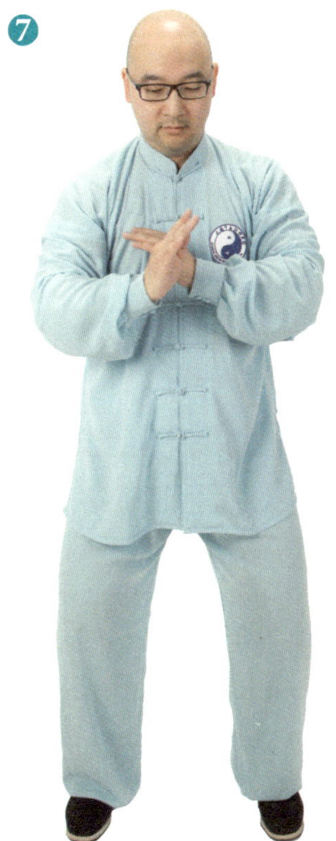

7. Close the hands in front of the chest again.

8. Clench fists and close them on both sides of the lower abdomen.

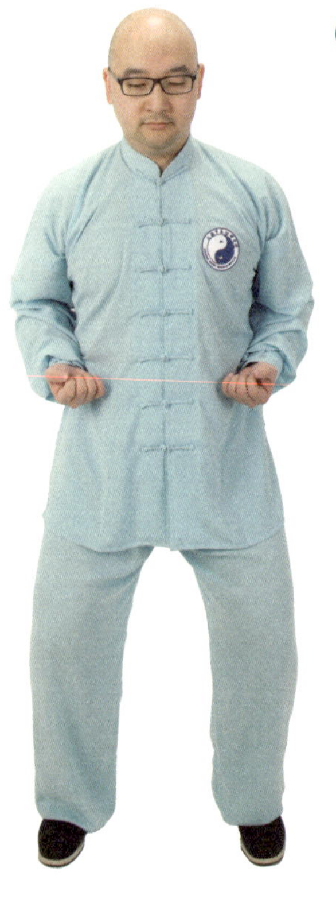

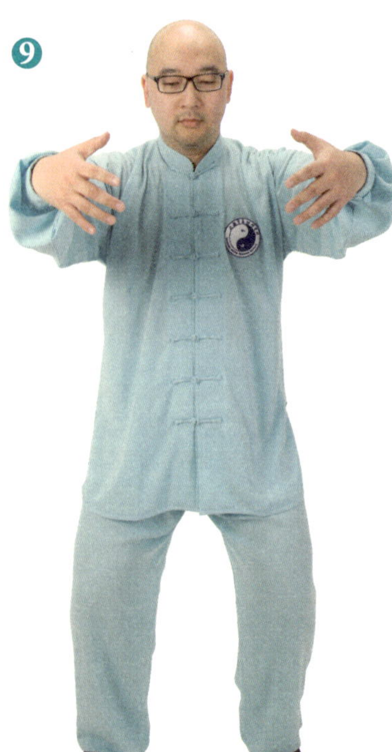

9. Return to standing posture with imagination of holding a ball: Place your feet shoulder-width apart, slightly bend your knees and do not let your knees go past your toes, and raise your arms to the level of your chest.

Movement Two: Draw the Bow Both Left and Right-Handed to Shoot the Hawk

About this movement: This movement focuses on the opening and closing of *qi* activity, especially on three acupoints: Danzhong (CV 17)[1] , Shenque (CV 8)[2] and Qihai (CV 6)[3]. Arm extension, chest expansion and neck rotation strengthen muscles in the shoulder, arm, neck and rib-side area and benefit *qi* and blood circulation of the heart and lung.

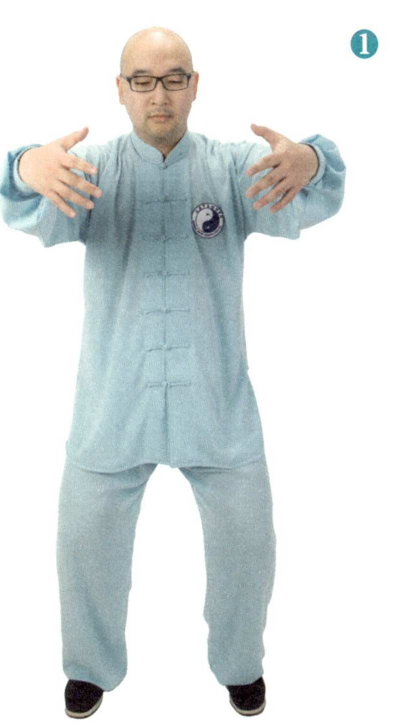

1. Standing posture with imagination of holding a ball: Place your feet shoulder-width apart, slightly bend your knees and do not let your knees go past your toes, and raise your arms to the level of your chest.

1 An acupuncture point located in the thorax, at the midpoint between the nipples, horizontally at the 4th intercostal space.

2 An acupuncture point located in the center of the umbilicus.

3 An acupuncture point located in the lower abdomen, on the anterior midline, 1.5 cun (about 2-finger width) below the umbilicus.

2. Turn to the right side, touch the floor with the right tiptoe, and place the body weight on the left foot. Raise your arms to the level of your chest with imagination of holding a ball.

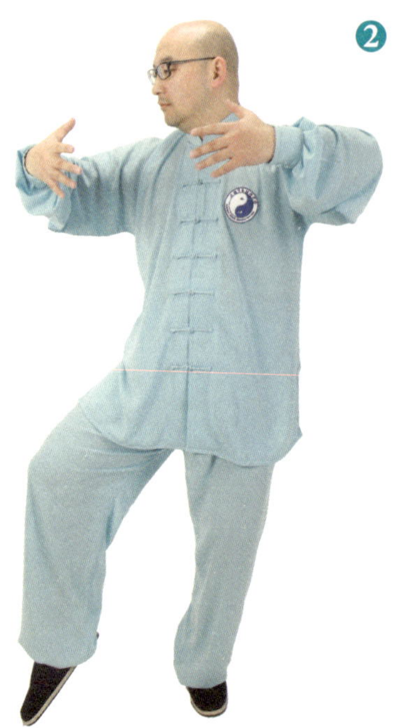

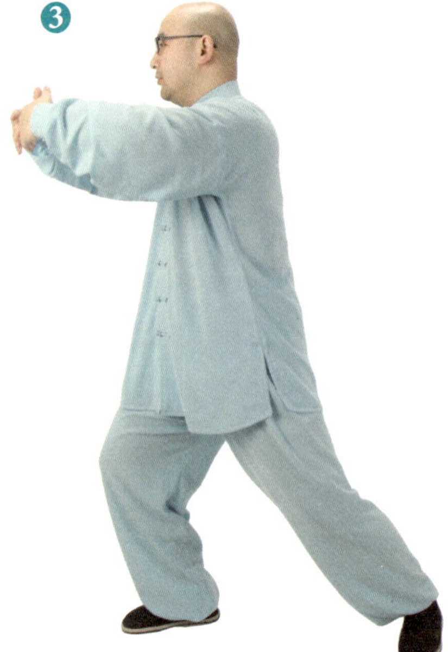

3. Touch the floor with the right foot, shift the body weight to the right foot first and then to the left foot. Lift the hands and close them in front of the chest and shift the body weight to the right foot again.

4. Shift the body weight to the left foot again. Extend the hands forward from the chest and shift the body weight to the right foot.

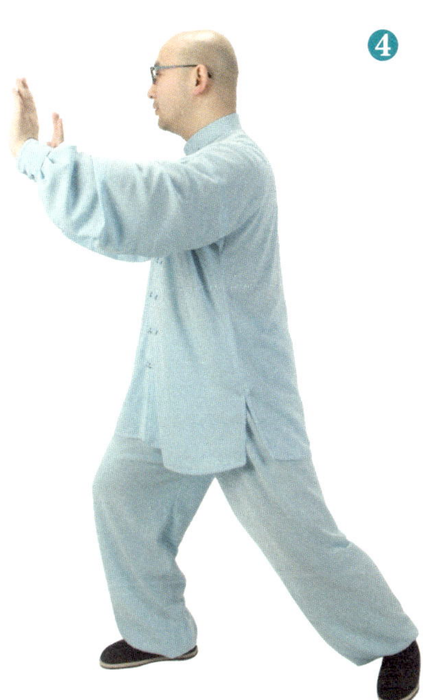

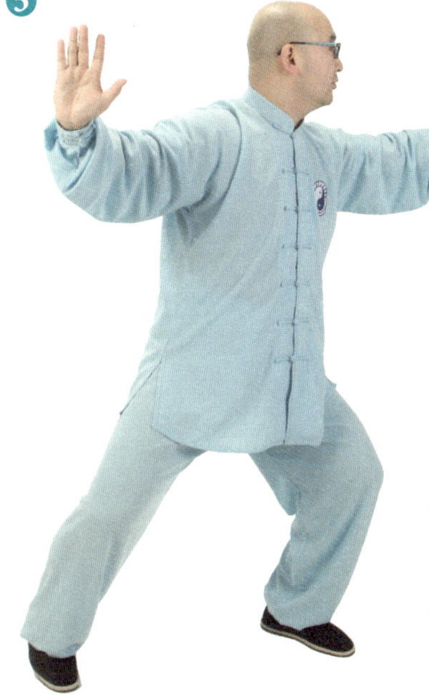

5. Shift the body weight to the right foot, turn 180° to the left. Draw a downward arc using the left hand and extend forward from left side of the body.

6. Draw downward arcs using both hands and cross the hands in front of the chest.

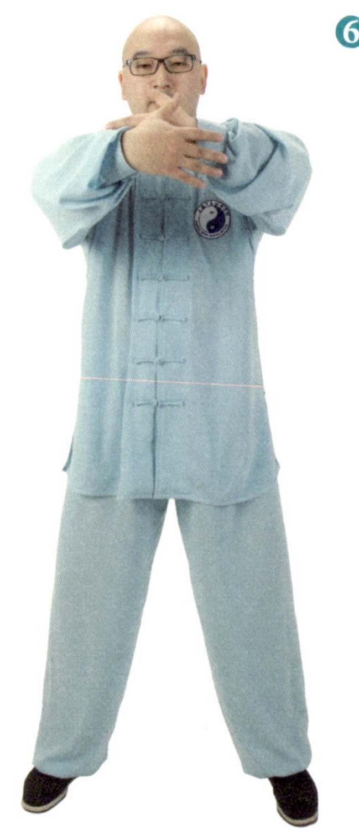

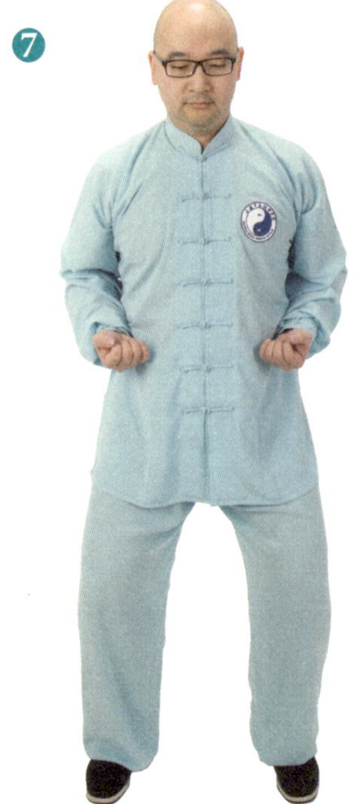

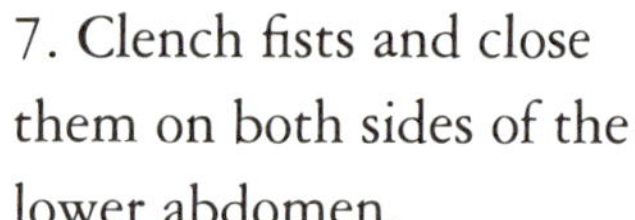

7. Clench fists and close them on both sides of the lower abdomen.

8. Return to standing posture with imagination of holding a ball: Place your feet shoulder-width apart, slightly bend your knees and do not let your knees go past your toes, and raise your arms to the level of your chest.

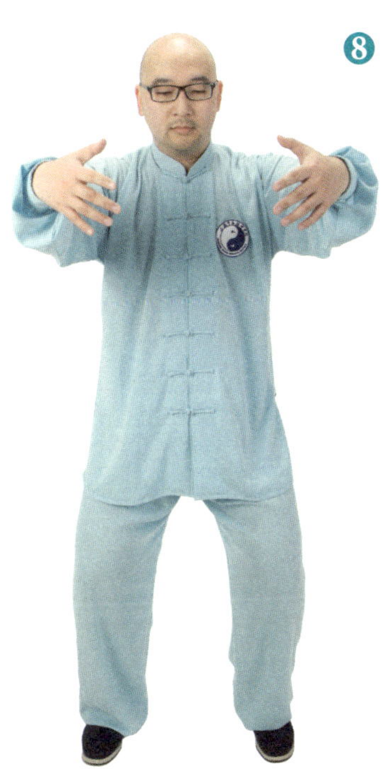

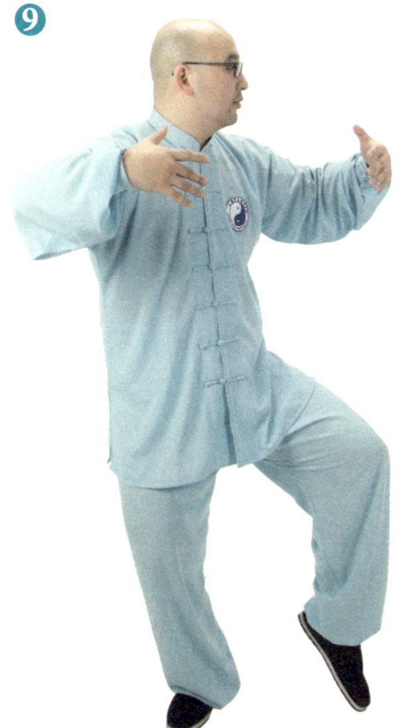

9. Turn to the left, touch the floor with the left tiptoe and place the body weight on the right foot. Raise your arms to the level of your chest with imagination of holding a ball.

10. Touch the floor with the left foot, shift the body weight to the left foot first and then to the right foot. Lift the hands and close them in front of the chest and shift the body weight to the left foot again.

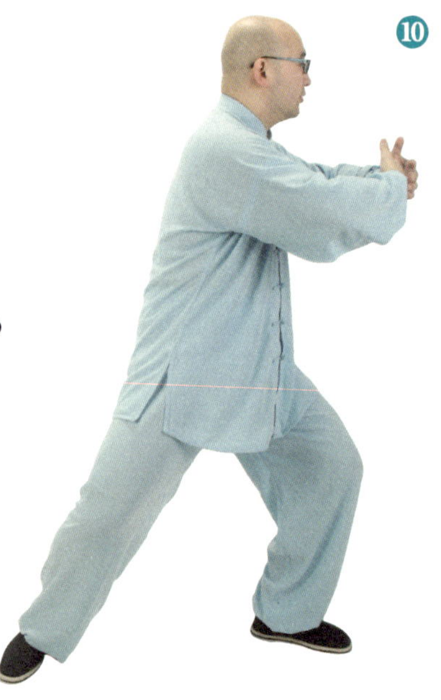

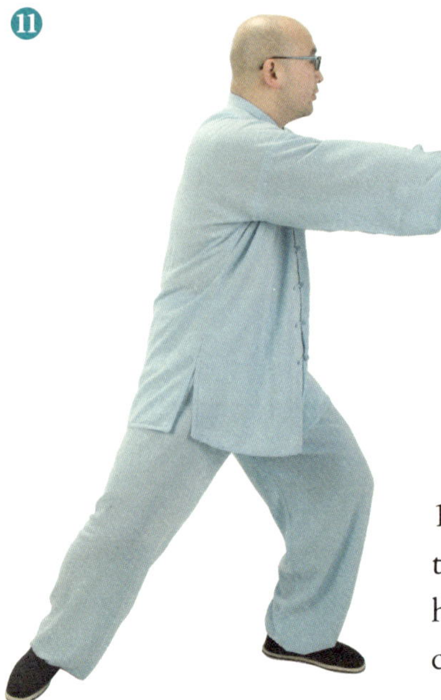

11. Shift the body weight to the right foot extend the hands forward from the chest and shift the body weight to the left foot.

12. After shifting the body weight to the left foot, turn 180° to the right. Draw a downward arc using the right hand and extend forward from right side of the body.

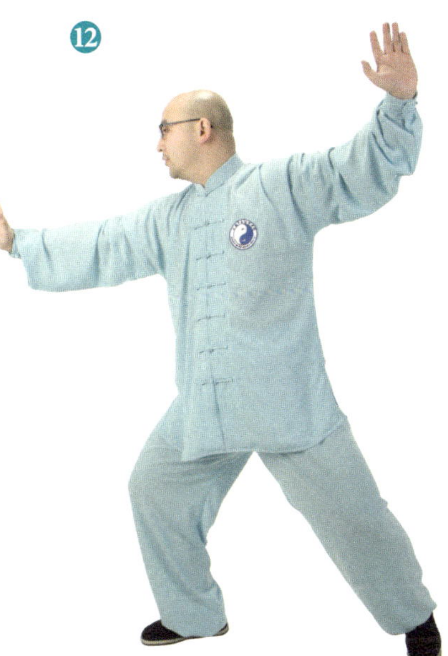

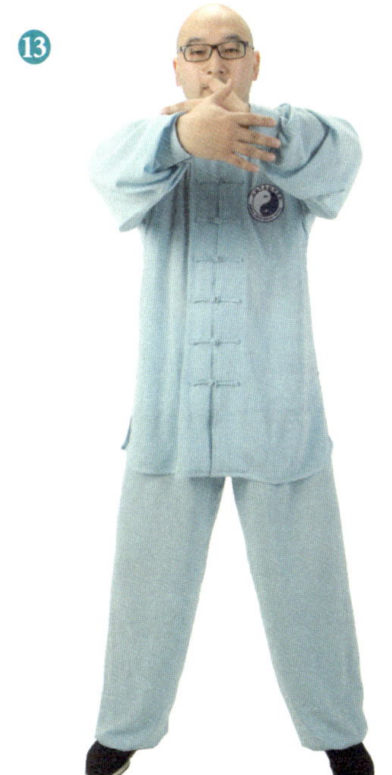

13. Draw downward arcs using both hands and cross the hands in front of the chest.

14. Clench fists and put them on both sides of the lower abdomen.

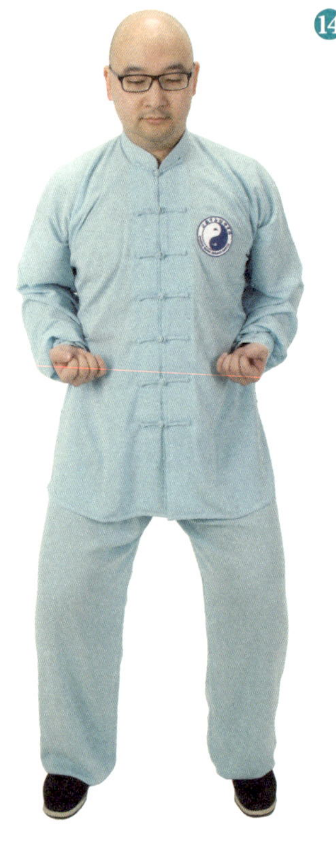

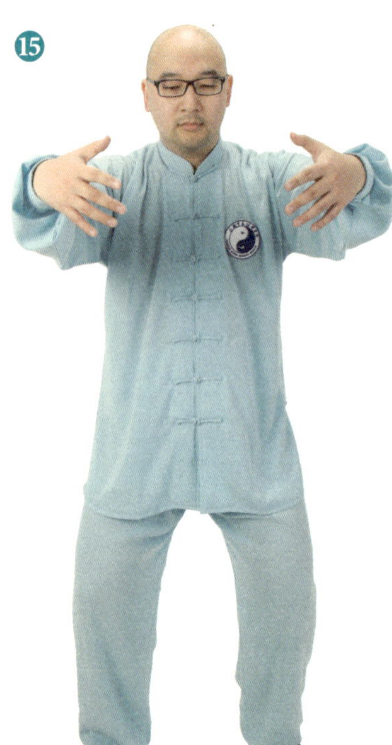

15. Return to standing posture with imagination of holding a ball: Place your feet shoulder-width apart, slightly bend your knees and do not let your knees go past your toes, and raise your arms to the level of your chest.

Movement Three: Hold One Arm Aloft to Regulate the Spleen and Stomach

About the movement: This movement mainly emphasizes the ascending and descending of *qi*, forming left and right rotations of its flow. By upward and downward rotation, this movement can influence muscles on both sides and internal organs including the liver, gallbladder, spleen and stomach, thus increasing the gastrointestinal peristalsis and improving digestion.

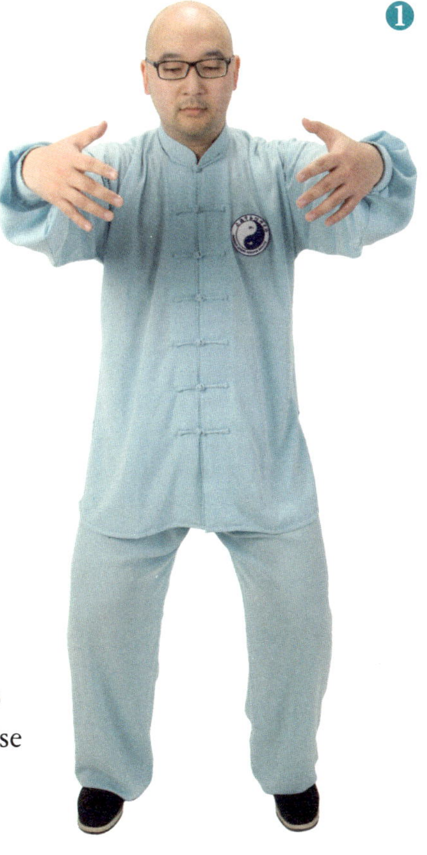

1. Standing posture with imagination of holding a ball: Place your feet shoulder-width apart, slightly bend your knees and do not let your knees go past your toes, and raise your arms to the level of your chest.

2. Shift to standing posture with imagination of holding a ball longitudinally, with left hand on top and right hand down. Place the body weight on the left foot.

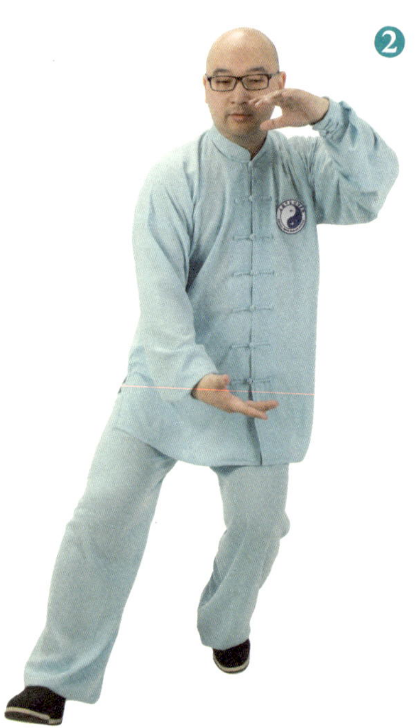

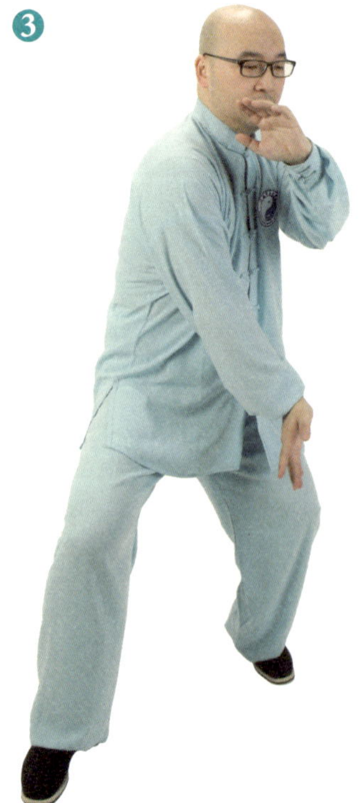

3. Cross the hands, repeat three times and gradually enlarge the ball in imagination.

4. Lift the right hand, press the left hand down.

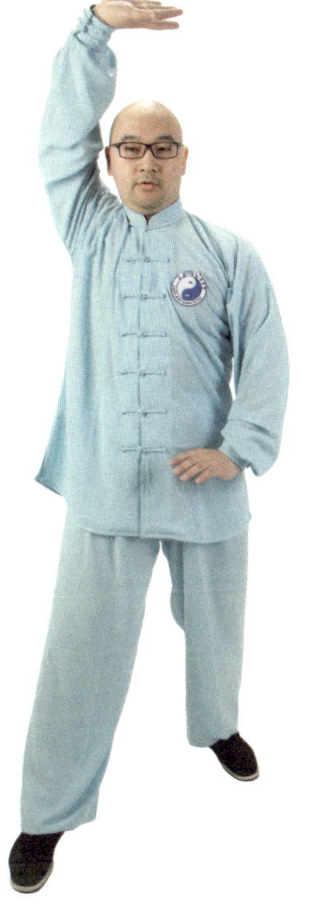

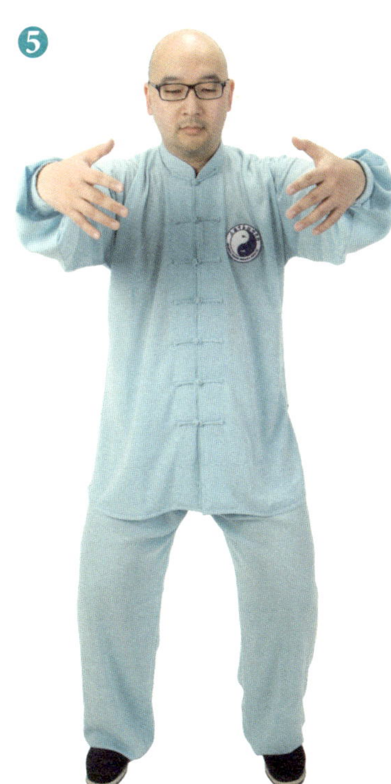

5. Return to standing posture with imagination of holding a ball: Place your feet shoulder-width apart, slightly bend your knees and do not let your knees go past your toes, and raise your arms to the level of your chest.

6. Shift to standing posture with imagination of holding a ball longitudinally, with right hand on top and left hand down. Place the body weight on the right foot.

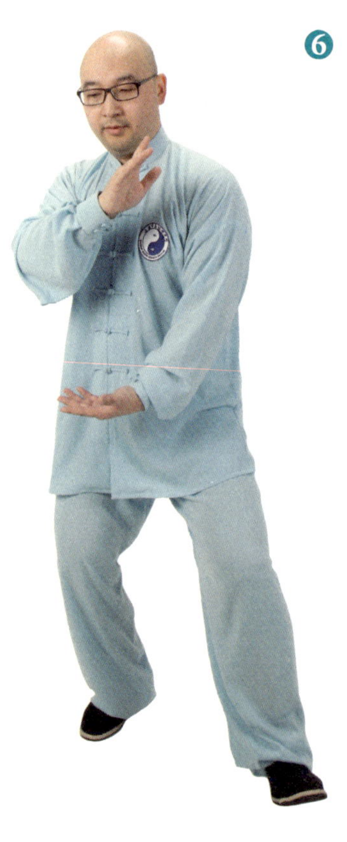

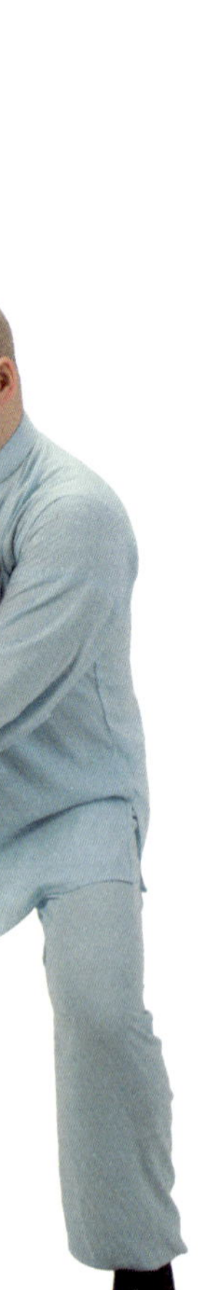

7. Cross hands, repeat three times and gradually enlarge the ball in imagination.

8. Lift the left hand, press the right hand down.

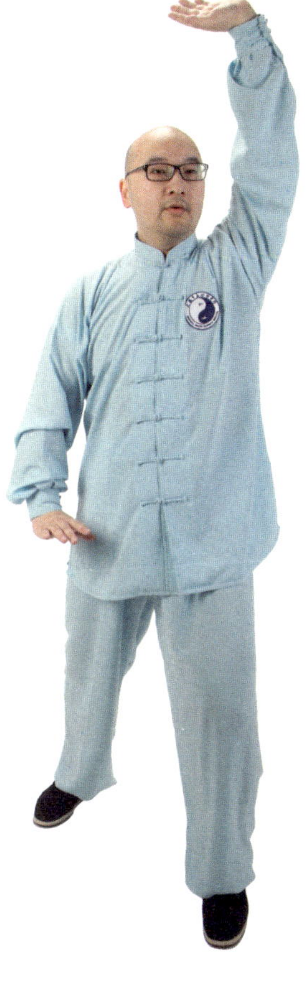

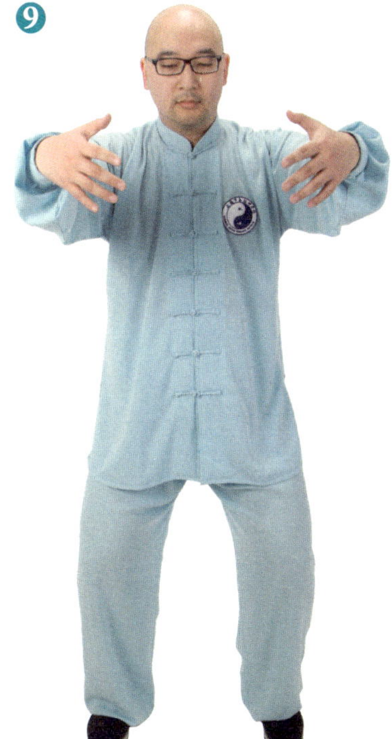

9. Return to standing posture with imagination of holding a ball: Place your feet shoulder-width apart, slightly bend your knees and do not let your knees go past your toes, and raise your arms to the level of your chest.

Movement Four: Look from Side to Side to Prevent Five Overstrains and Seven Injuries

About the movement: This movement focuses on spiral circling of *qi* activity. By working on the spine and thighs, it helps to regulate functions of the nervous system, improve fatigue and harmonize *qi* and blood. This movement also helps to prevent and treat hypertension, cervical spondylosis and eye problems.

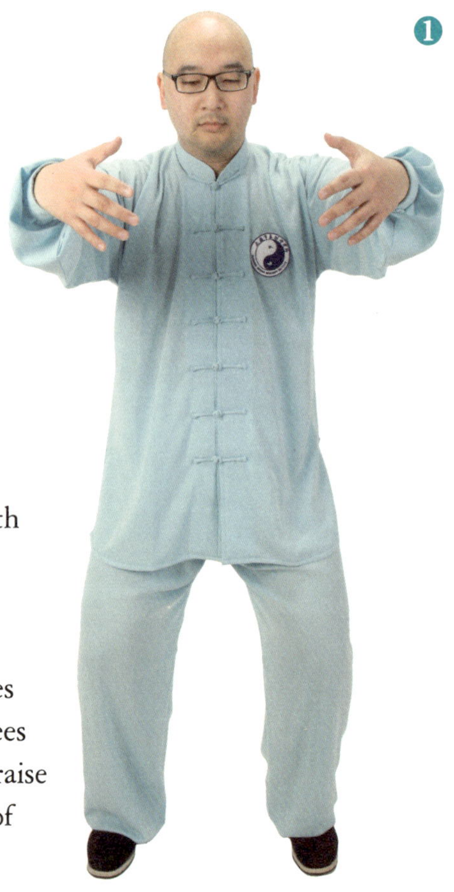

1. Standing posture with imagination of holding a ball: Place your feet shoulder-width apart, slightly bend your knees and do not let your knees go past your toes, and raise your arms to the level of your chest.

2. Move the right foot 45° backward and turn the hands like rolling a ball.

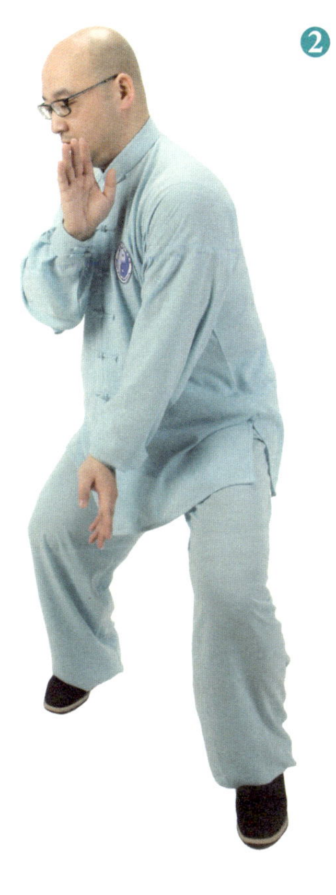

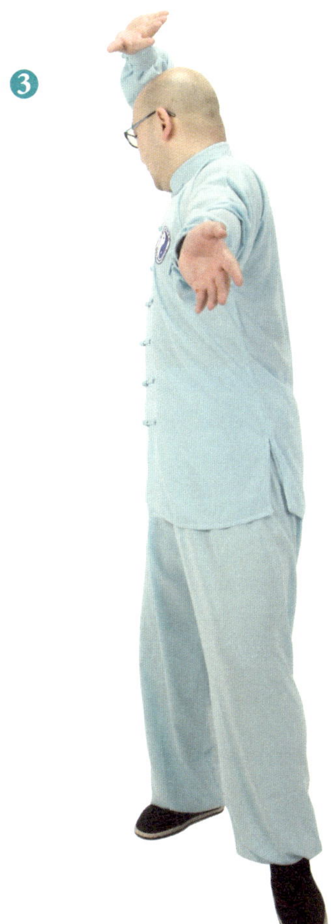

3. Turn your body to the right and back, lifting both hands like holding a ball.

4. Squat down and turn left, dropping both hands like holding a ball.

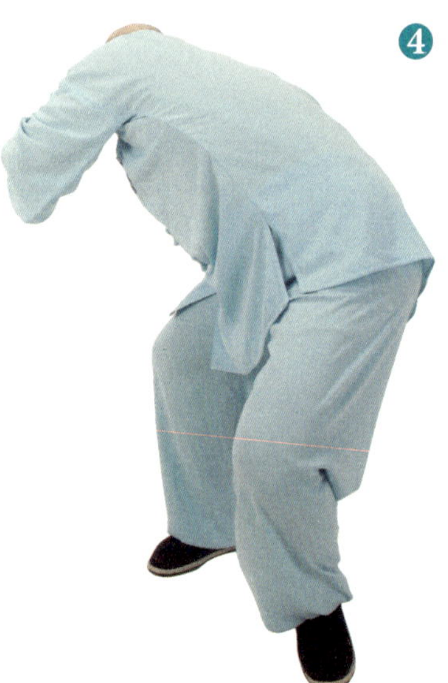

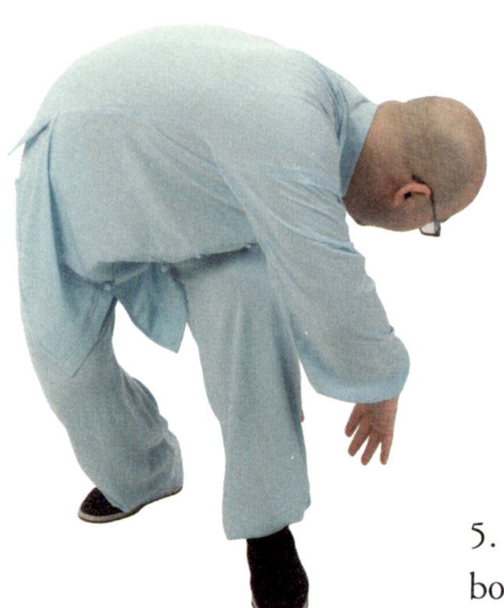

5. Continue to turn the body to the left until the back of the left foot. Dropping both hands like holding a ball.

6. Turn the body upright and lift the hands like holding a ball.

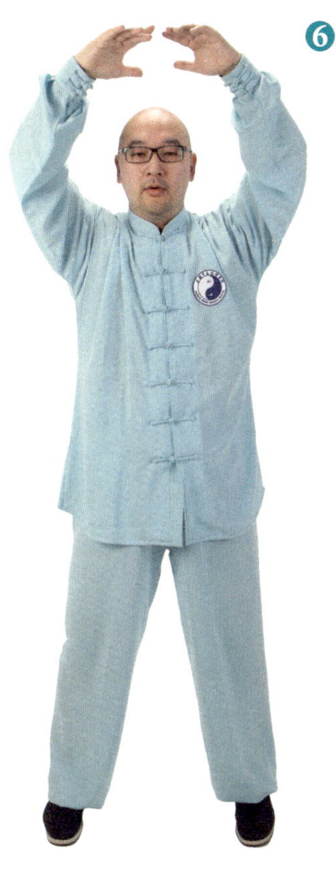

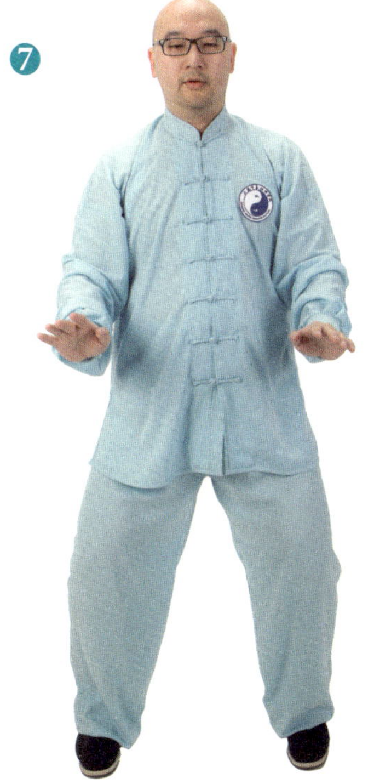

7. Slowly drop the hands like holding a ball.

8. Shift the body weight to the left side, move the left foot to right, open the hands and drop the right hand to the lateral side of the right leg. Drop the right hand along the lateral side of the right leg, shift the body weight to the right side.

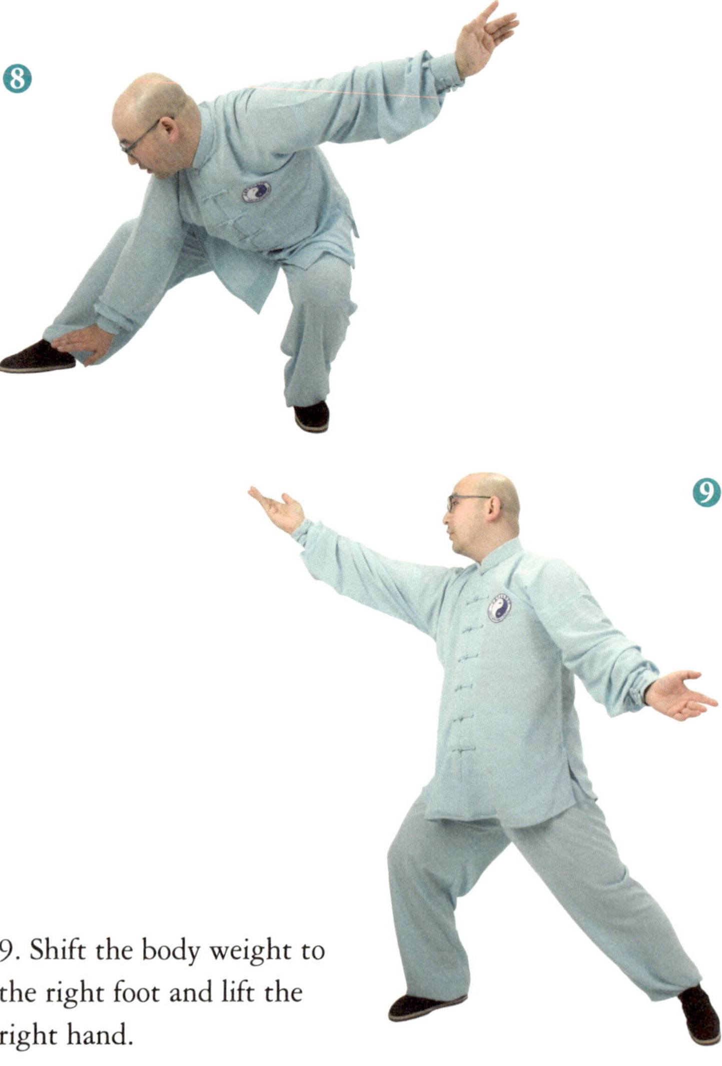

9. Shift the body weight to the right foot and lift the right hand.

10. Turn the body to the left, drop the left hand along the lateral side of the left leg and shift the body weight to the left side.

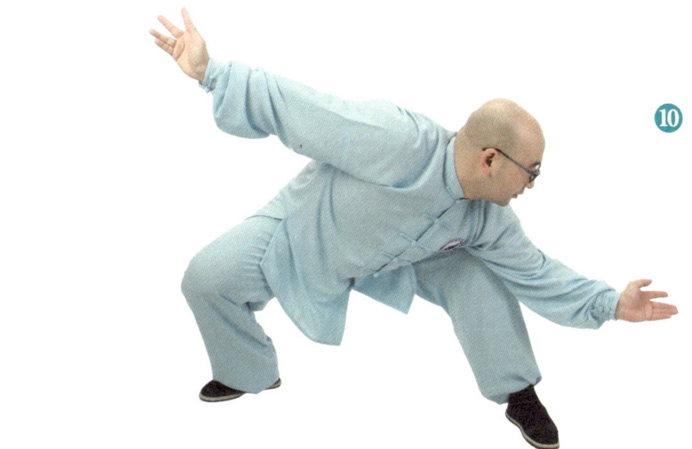

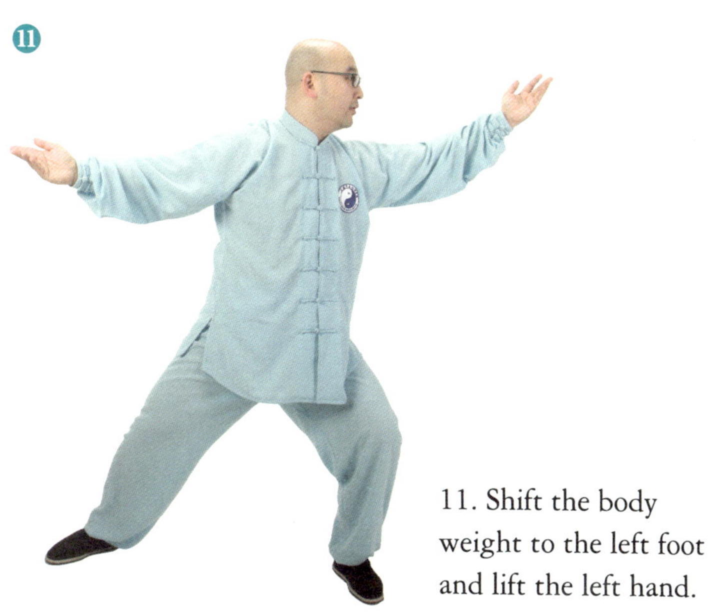

11. Shift the body weight to the left foot and lift the left hand.

12. Return to standing posture with imagination of holding a ball: Place your feet shoulder-width apart, slightly bend your knees and do not let your knees go past your toes, and raise your arms to the level of your chest.

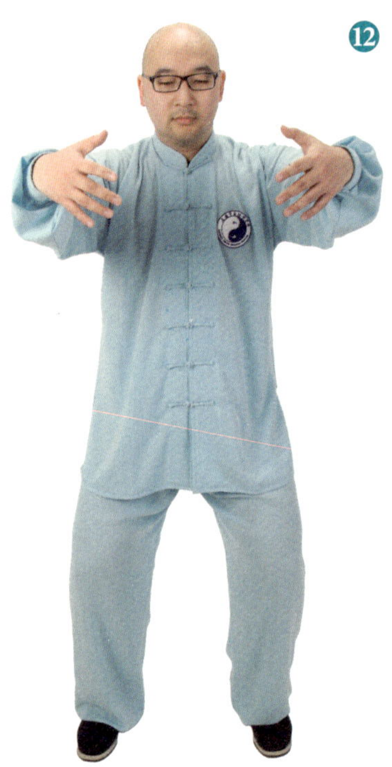

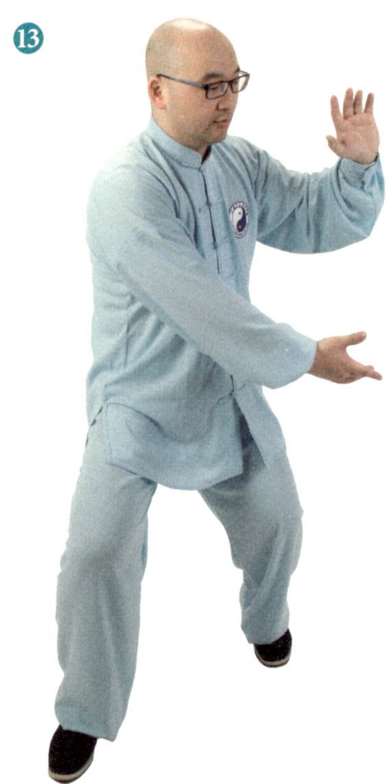

13. Move the left foot 45° backward and turn the hands like rolling a ball.

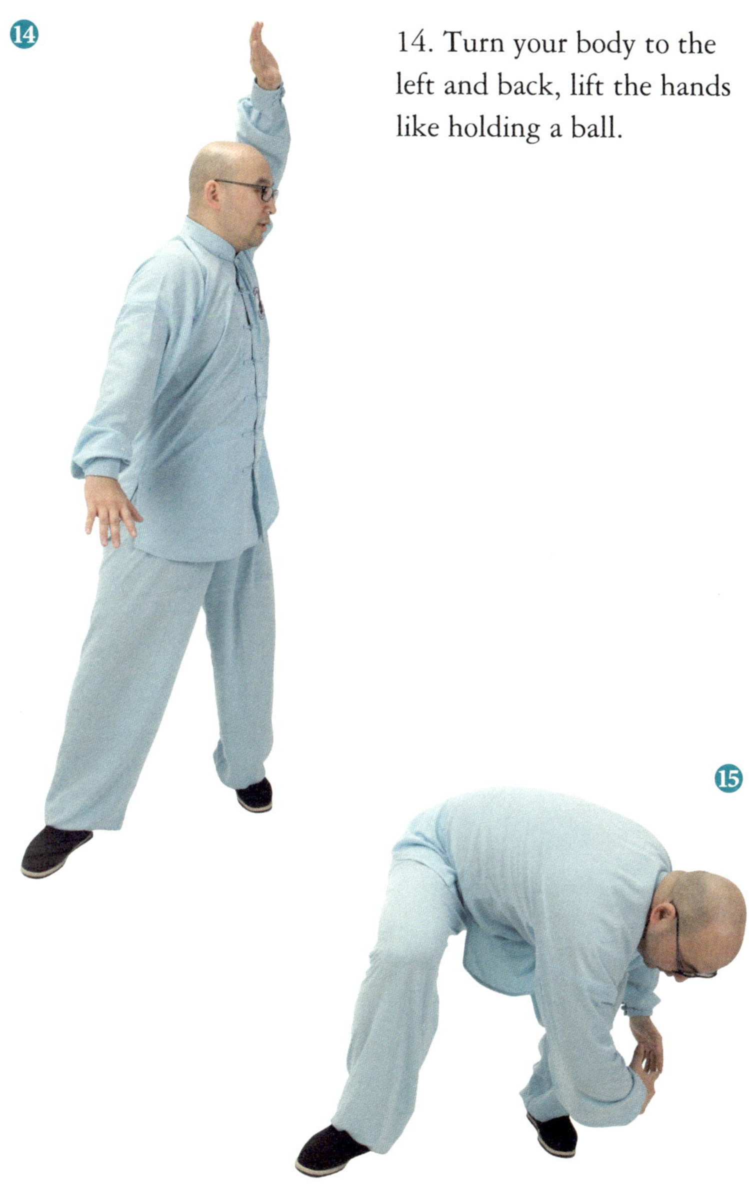

14. Turn your body to the left and back, lift the hands like holding a ball.

15. Squat down and turn right, drop the hands like holding a ball.

16. Continue turning the body to the right until the back of the right foot and drop the hands like holding a ball.

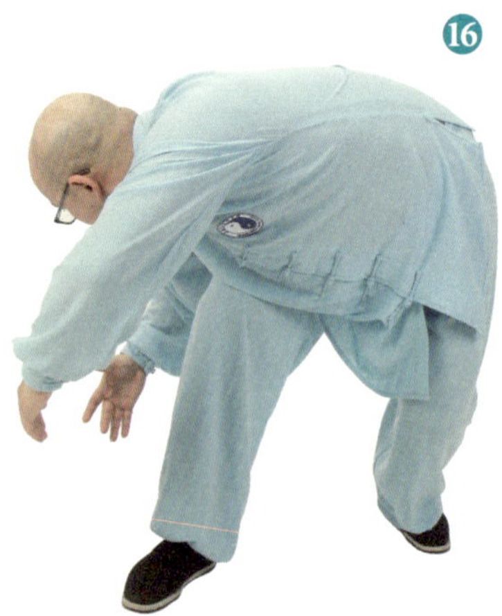

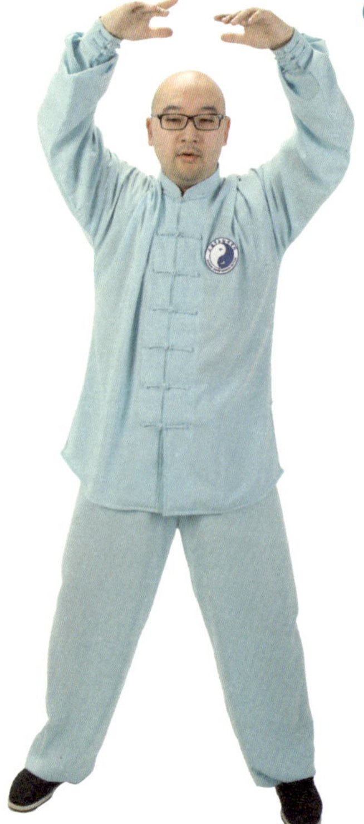

17. Turn the body upright and lift the hands like holding a ball.

18. Slowly drop the hands like holding a ball.

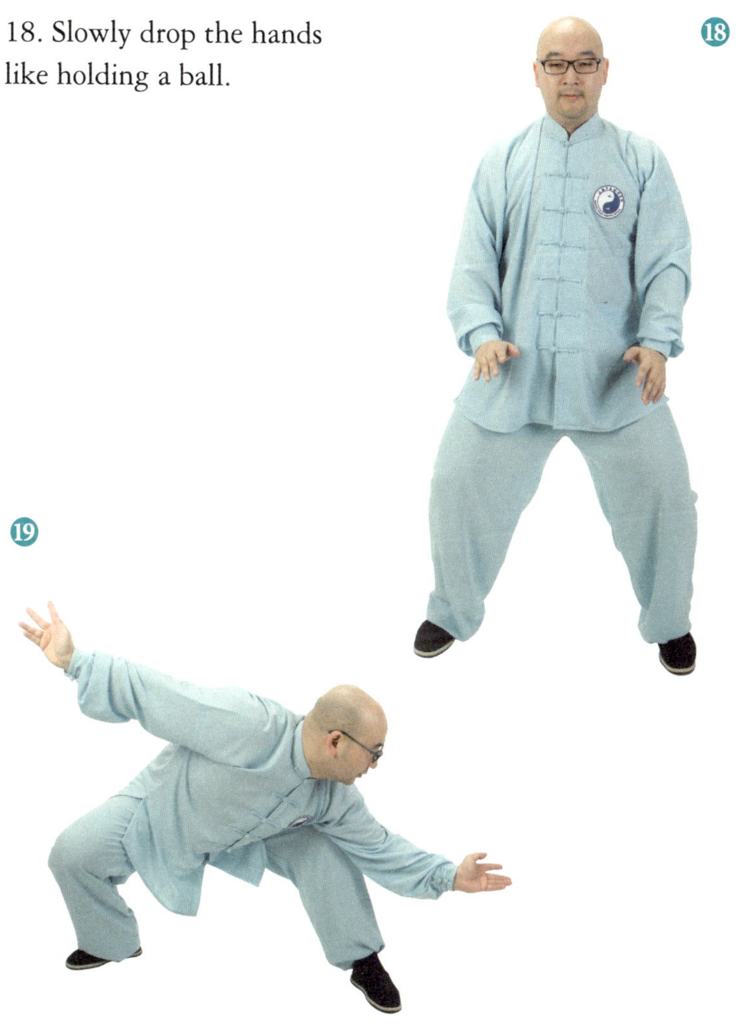

19. Shift the body weight to the right side, move the right foot to the left, open the hands and then place the left hand down to the lateral side of the left leg. Drop the left hand along the lateral side of the left leg and shift the body weight to the left side.

20. Shift the body weight to the left foot and lift the left hand.

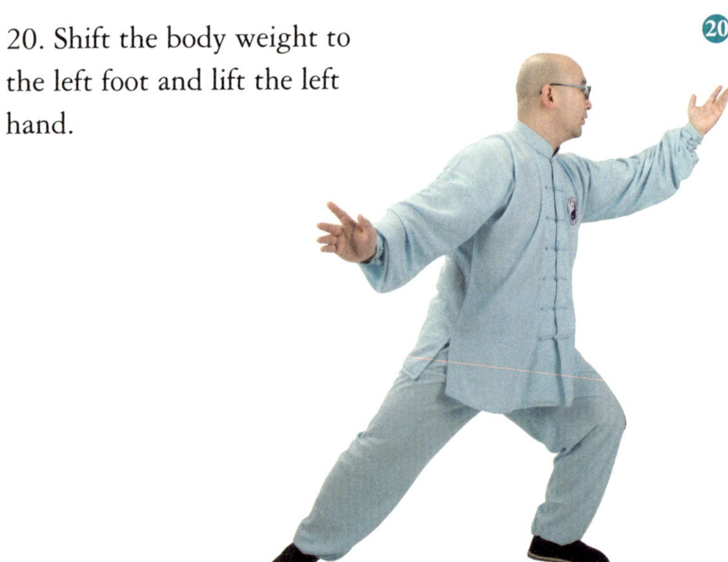

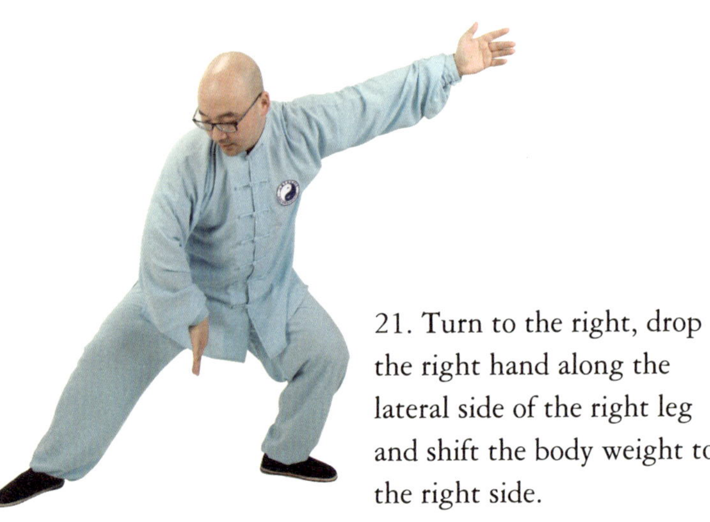

21. Turn to the right, drop the right hand along the lateral side of the right leg and shift the body weight to the right side.

22. Shift the body weight to the right foot and lift the right hand.

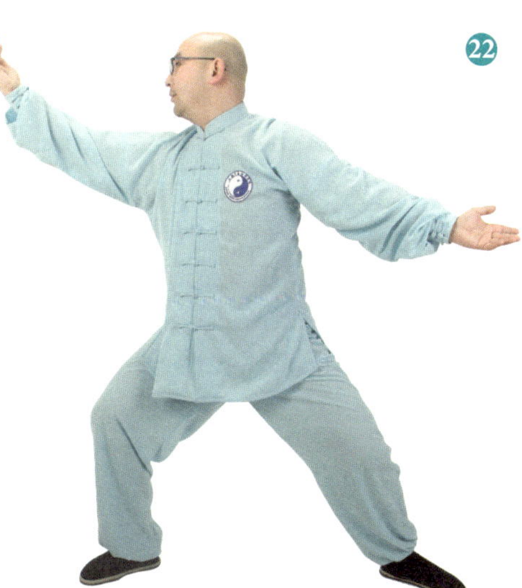

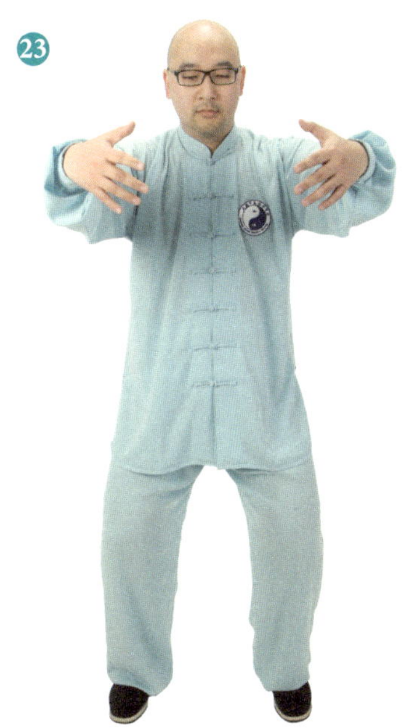

23. Return to standing posture with imagination of holding a ball: Place your feet shoulder-width apart, slightly bend your knees and do not let your knees go past your toes, and raise your arms to the level of your chest.

Movement Five: Sway the Head and Shake to Clear Heart-Fire

About the movement: This movement focuses on *qi* sinking down to Dantian and restrain *qi* within bones. By exercising lumbar and cervical joints, this movement can regulate *qi* circulation in the Conception, Governor and Throughfare Vessels and harmonize heart fire and kidney water. It can also prevent or treat neck back, low back pain and problems due to heart-fire hyperactivity such as insomnia, restlessness and palpitations.

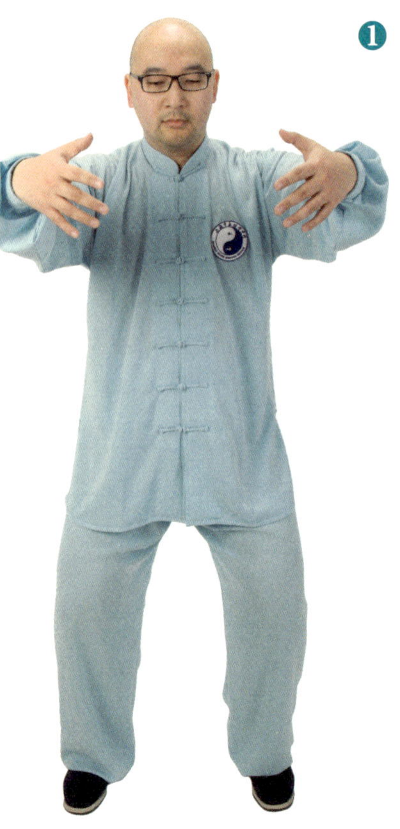

1. Standing posture with imagination of holding a ball: Place your feet shoulder-width apart, slightly bend your knees and do not let your knees go past your toes, and raise your arms to the level of your chest.

2. Move *qi* like moving the imaginary ball to turn the body to the right, slightly squatting down.

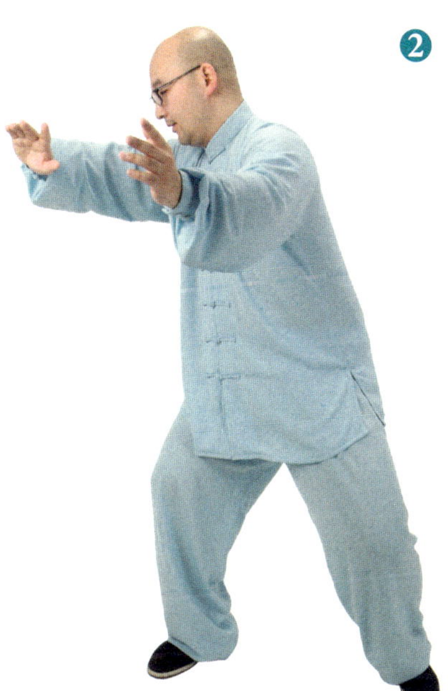

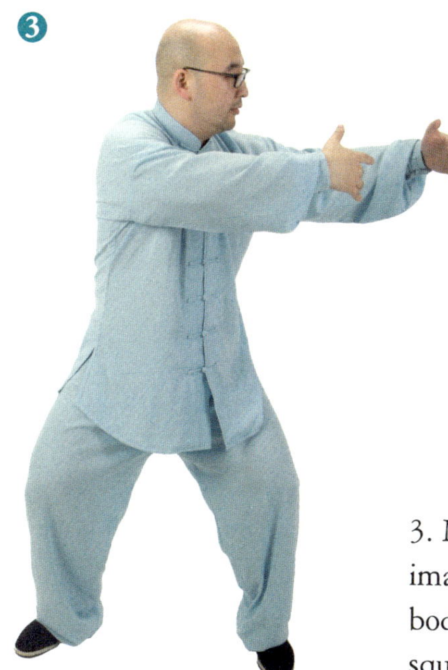

3. Move *qi* like moving the imaginary ball to turn the body to the left, slightly squatting down.

4. Move *qi* like moving the imaginary ball to turn the body to the right, slightly squatting down.

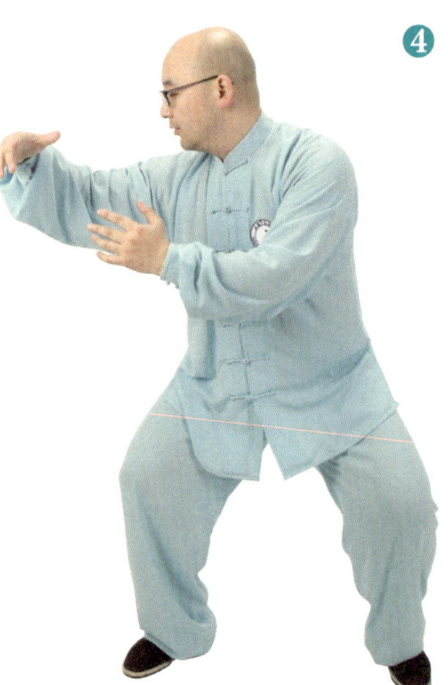

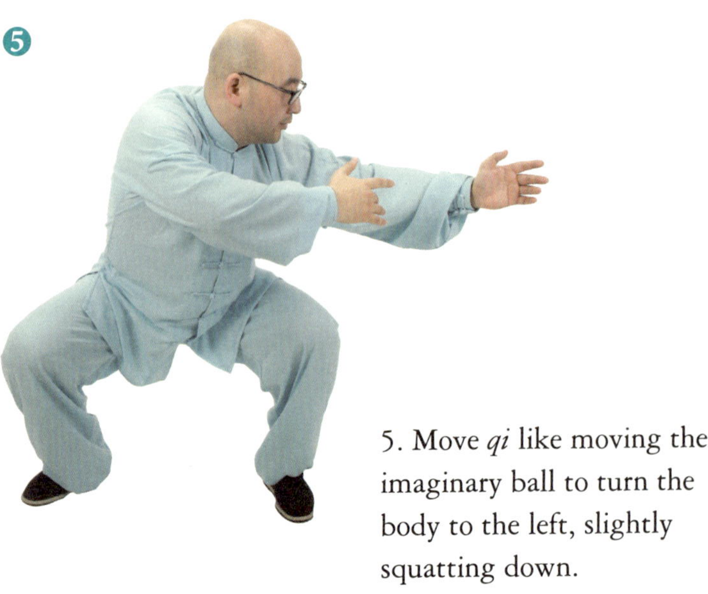

5. Move *qi* like moving the imaginary ball to turn the body to the left, slightly squatting down.

6. Move *qi* like moving the imaginary ball to turn the body to the right, slightly squatting down.

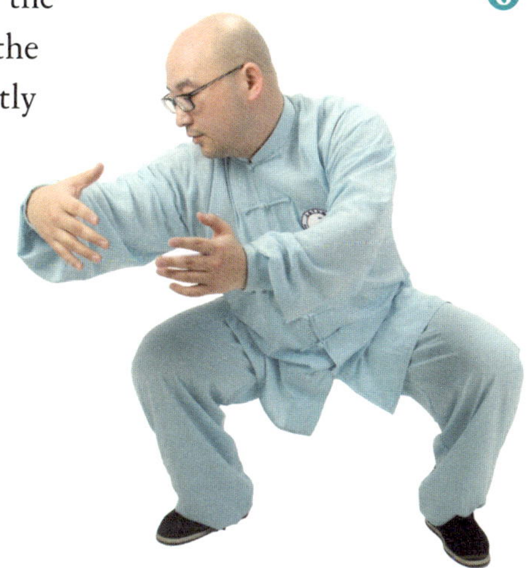

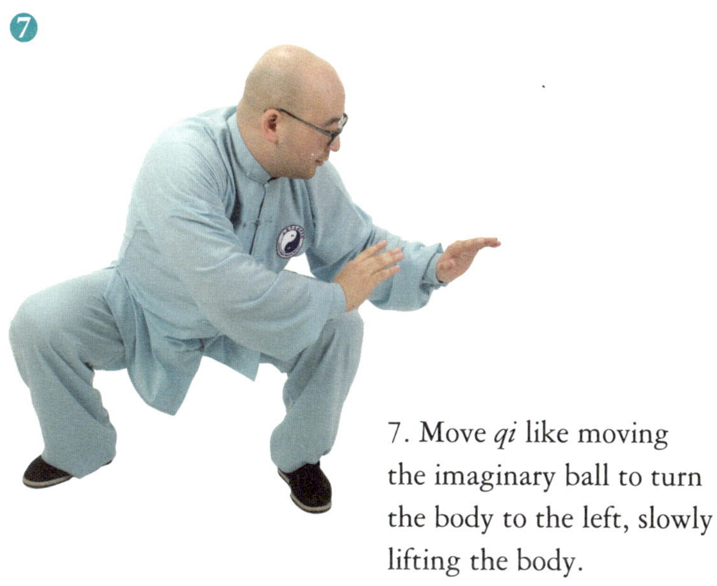

7. Move *qi* like moving the imaginary ball to turn the body to the left, slowly lifting the body.

8. Return to standing posture with imagination of holding a ball: Place your feet shoulder-width apart, slightly bend your knees and do not let your knees go past your toes, and raise your arms to the level of your chest.

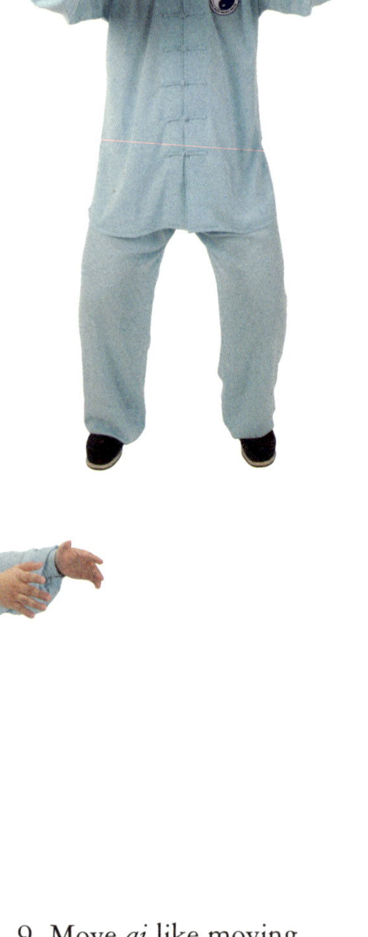

9. Move *qi* like moving the imaginary ball to turn the body to the left, slowly squatting down.

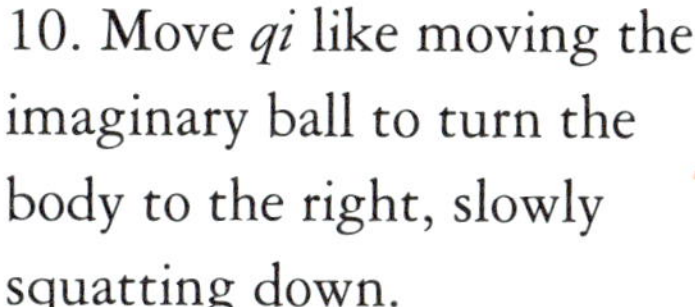

10. Move *qi* like moving the imaginary ball to turn the body to the right, slowly squatting down.

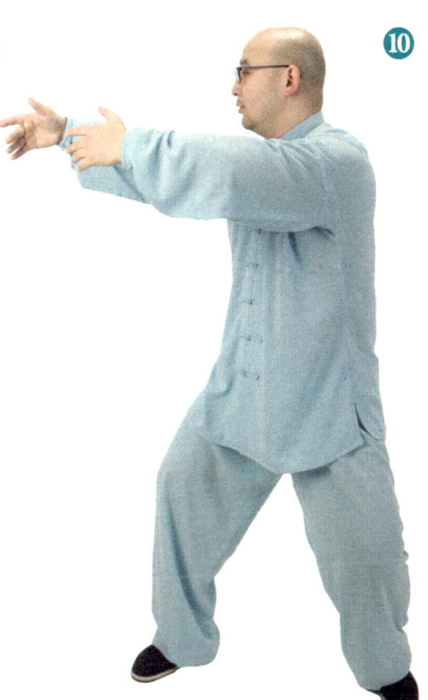

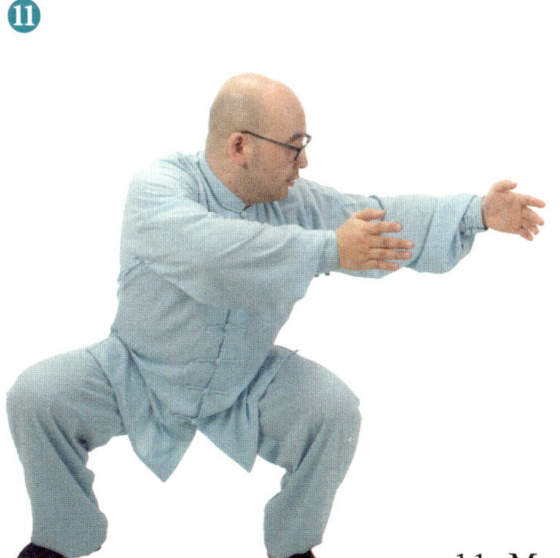

11. Move *qi* like moving the imaginary ball to turn the body to the left, slowly squatting down.

12. Move *qi* like moving the imaginary ball to turn the body to the right, slowly squatting down.

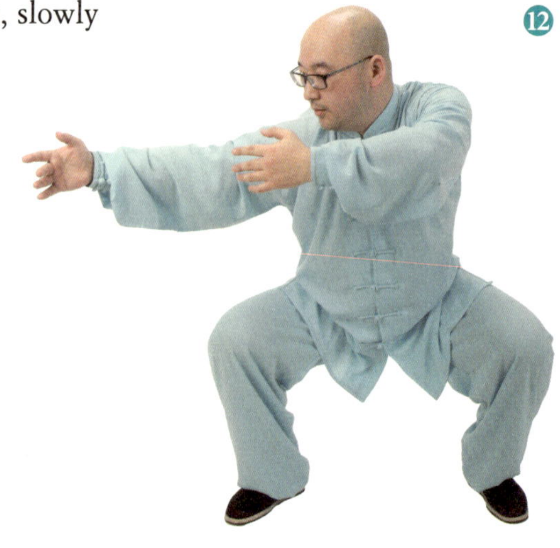

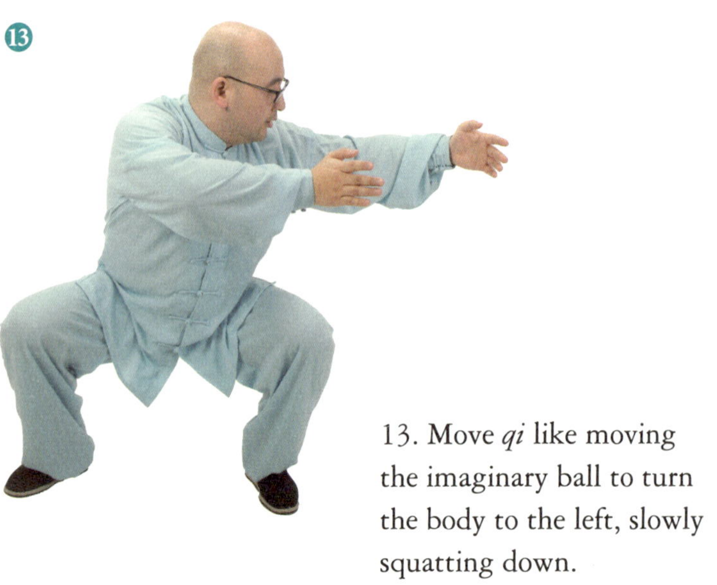

13. Move *qi* like moving the imaginary ball to turn the body to the left, slowly squatting down.

14. Move *qi* like moving the imaginary ball to turn the body to the right, slowly lifting the body.

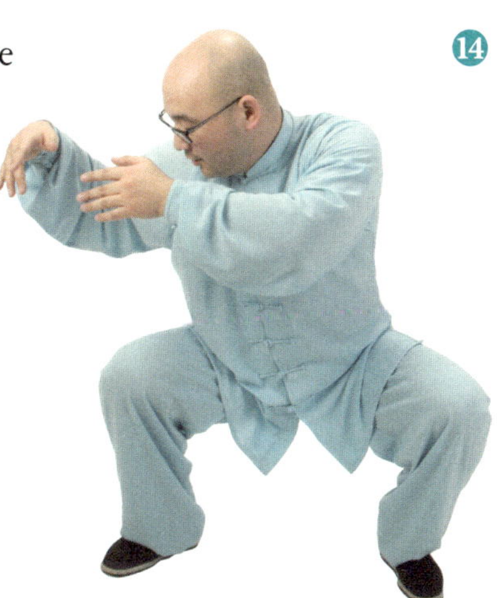

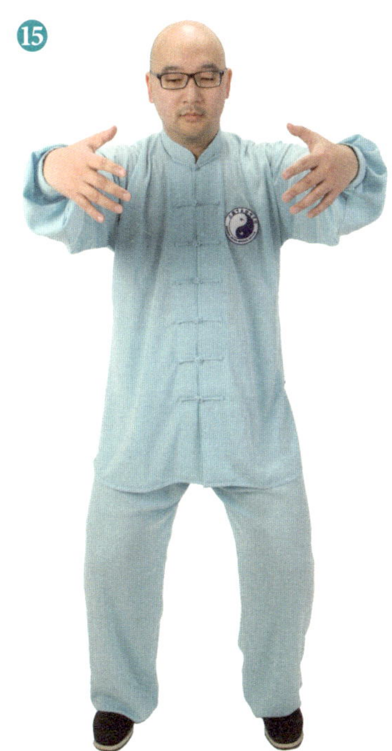

15. Return to standing posture with imagination of holding a ball: Place your feet shoulder-width apart, slightly bend your knees and do not let your knees go past your toes, and raise your arms to the level of your chest.

Movement Six: Hold the Feet with Both Hands to Consolidate the Kidney and Low Back

About the movement: This movement focuses on strengthening the real fire of the vital gate in the lumbus (known as the house of kidney). It can regulate the Belt, Conception, and Governor Vessels, benefit the kidney, refresh the mind and improve the eyesight.

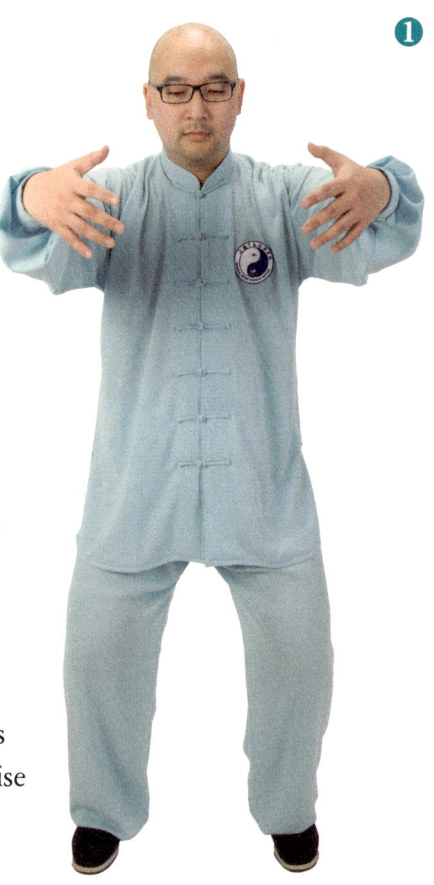

1. Standing posture with imagination of holding a ball: Place your feet shoulder-width apart, slightly bend your knees and do not let your knees go past your toes, and raise your arms to the level of your chest.

2. Lift both hands upward as if holding a ball, with the waist slightly arched backward and the chest rounded inward, as if embracing a ball.

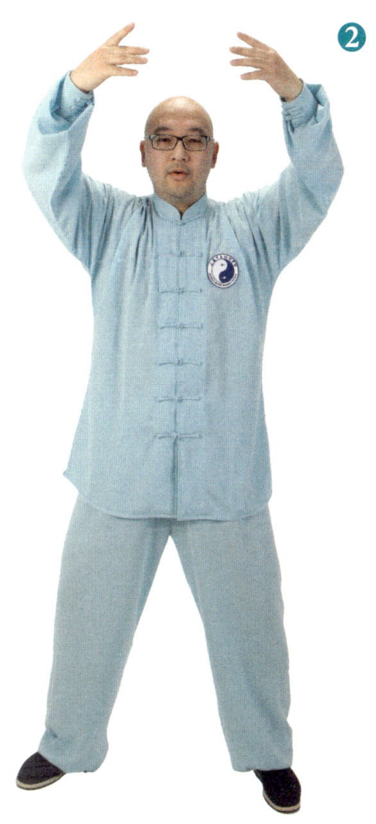

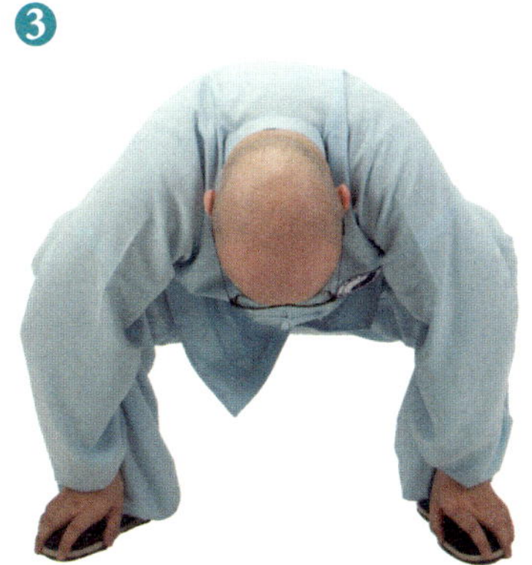

3. Bend the waist area and press the hands down on the top of your feet, like pressing a ball.

4. Move *qi* like moving a ball and gently lift the waist area.

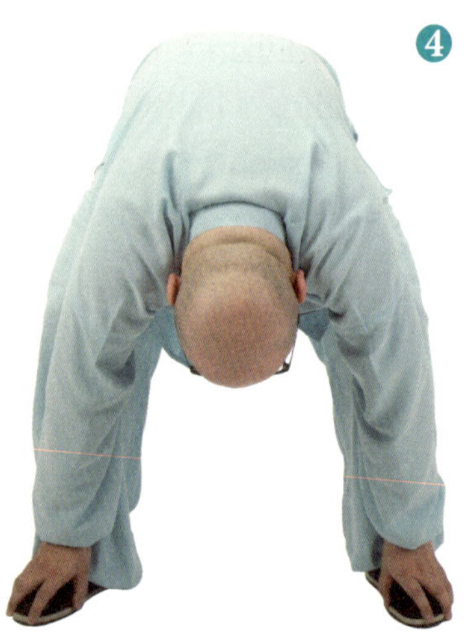

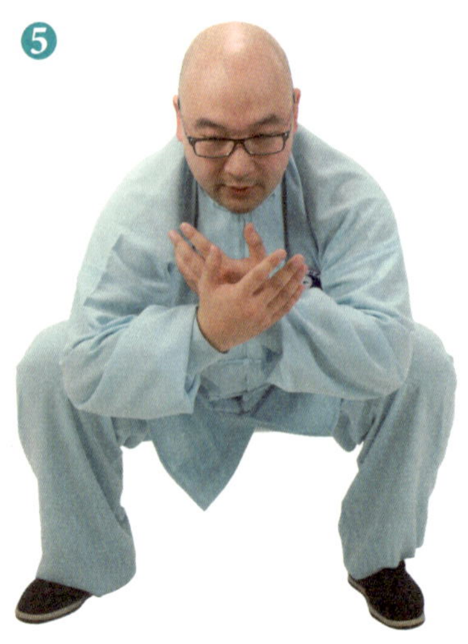

5. Move *qi* like moving a ball to the soles. Slowly drop the waist area.

6. Move *qi* liking moving a ball, gently support the low back and slowly lift the body.

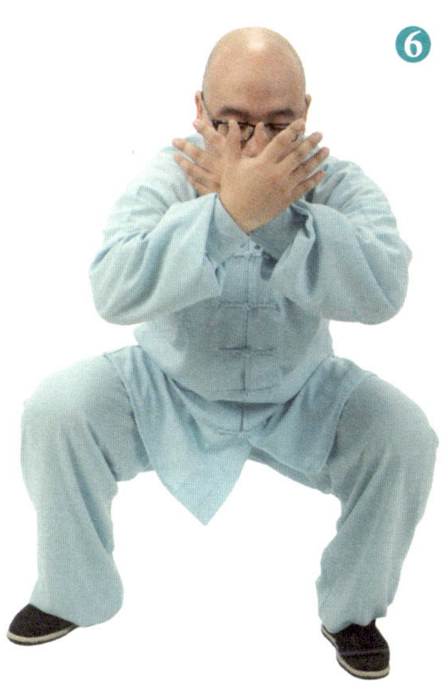

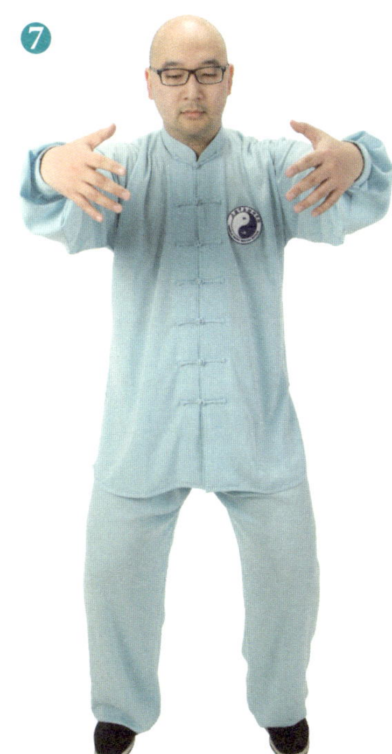

7. Return to standing posture with imagination of holding a ball: Place your feet shoulder-width apart, slightly bend your knees and do not let your knees go past your toes, and raise your arms to the level of your chest.

Movement Seven: Clench the Fists and Glare Angrily to Increase Strength

About the movement: This movement focuses on *qi* reaching the vertex, *qi* sinking down to Dantian and opening up and relaxing the hip joints. By excising muscles of the four limbs, low back and eyes, this movement can supplement lung *qi*, increase muscle strength and benefit sinews and bones.

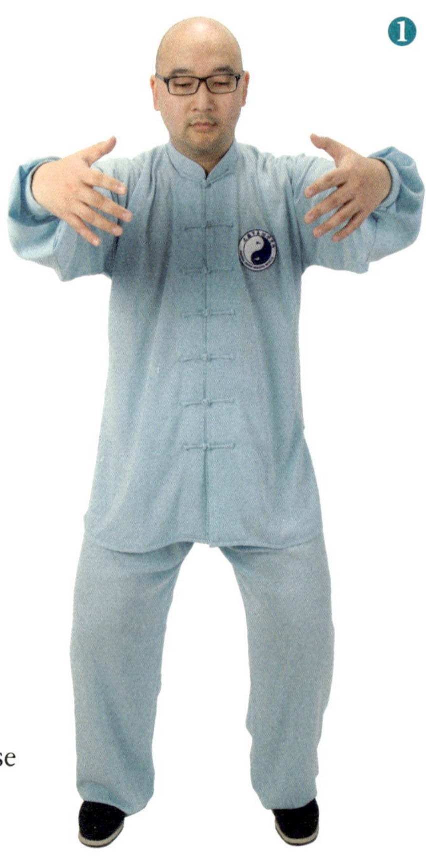

1. Standing posture with imagination of holding a ball: Place your feet shoulder-width apart, slightly bend your knees and do not let your knees go past your toes, and raise your arms to the level of your chest.

2. Move *qi* like moving a ball to turn the body to the right, place the body weight on the left foot, gently lift the right tiptoe and turn 45° to the right with the imagination of holding a ball.

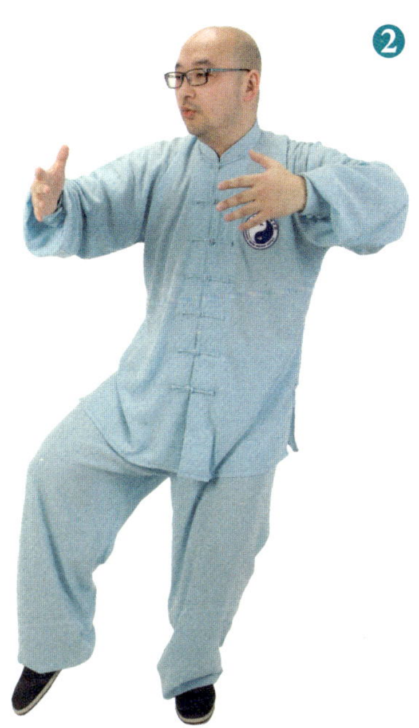

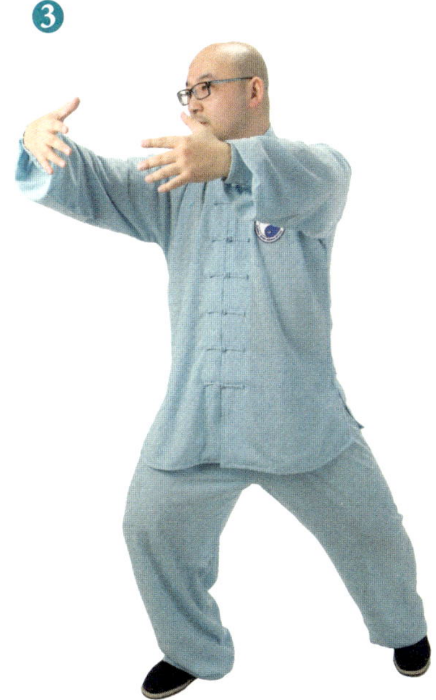

3. Move *qi* like moving a ball and turn 45° to the right and downward. Shift the body weight 45° forward to the right foot and hold the ball forward in the hands.

4. Move *qi* like moving a ball and turn inward and downward to shift the body weight to the left foot. Then use the hands to press the ball.

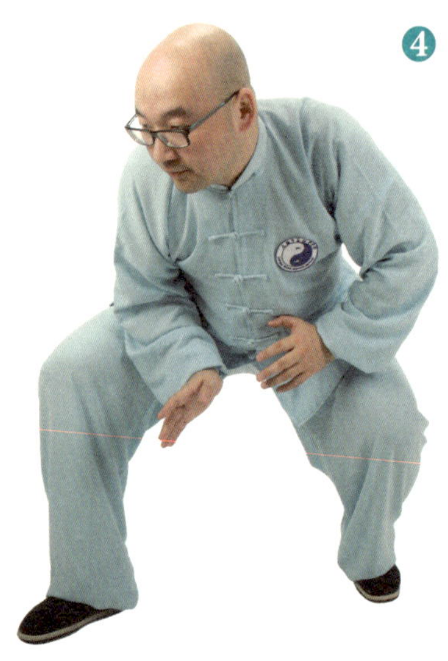

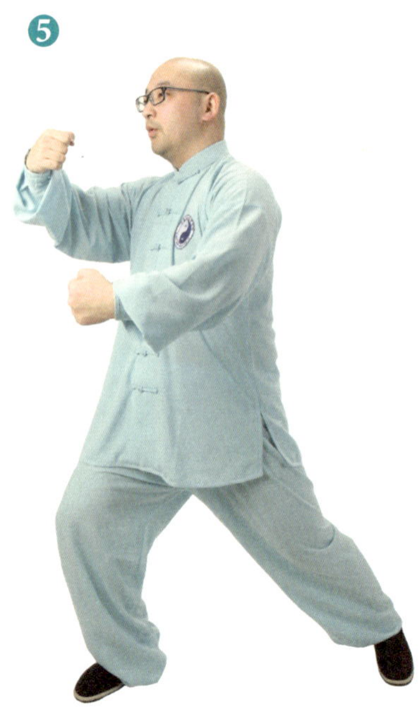

5. Move *qi* like moving a ball 45° upward and forward to shift the body weight to the right foot. Then punch with the fists. Allow your body and footwork to naturally follow the momentum of the punch without forcing any movement.

6. Return to standing posture with imagination of holding a ball: Place your feet shoulder-width apart, slightly bend your knees and do not let your knees go past your toes, and raise your arms to the level of your chest.

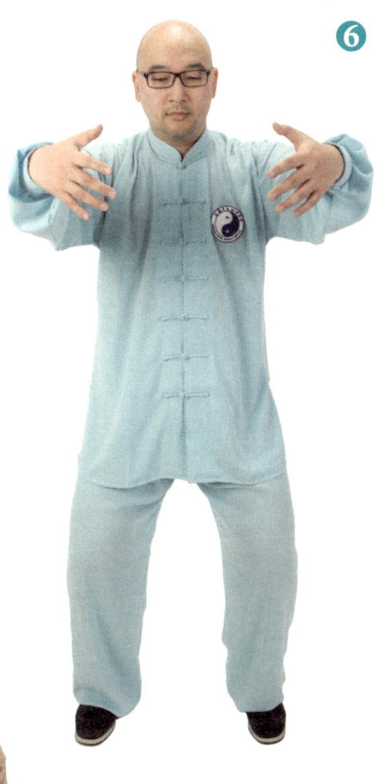

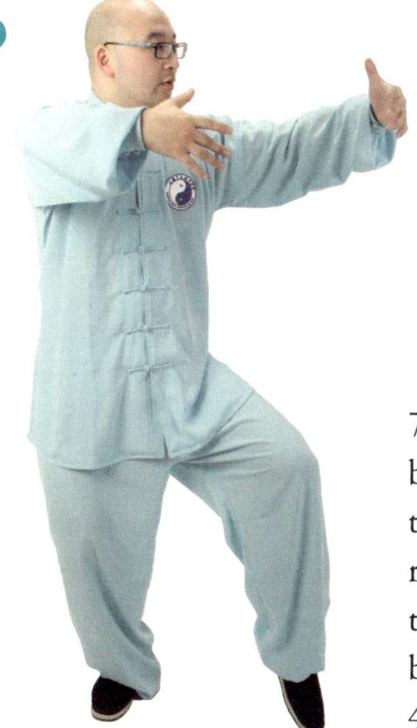

7. Move *qi* like moving a ball, turn to the left, place the body weight on the right foot and lift the left tiptoe. Hold the imaginary ball in the hands and turn 45° to the left side.

8. Move *qi* like moving a ball downward. Roll the ball 45° forward to shift the body weight 45° left and forward to the left foot. Hold the ball in the hands.

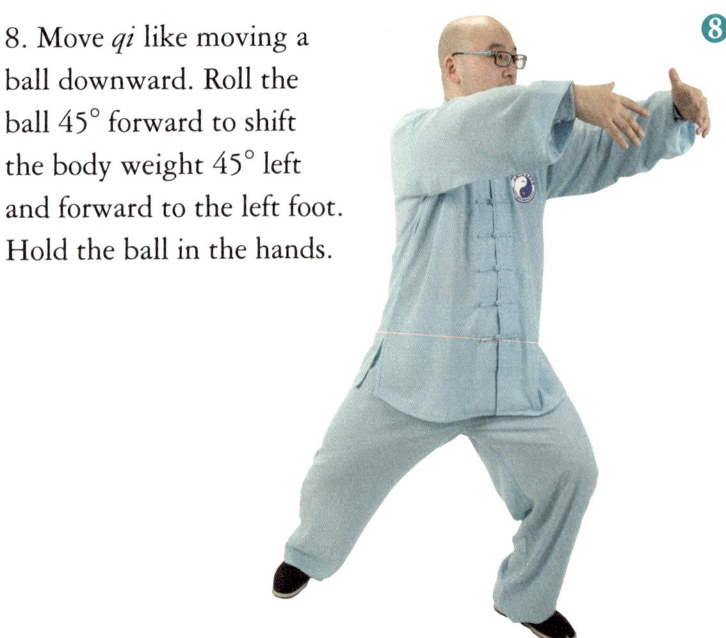

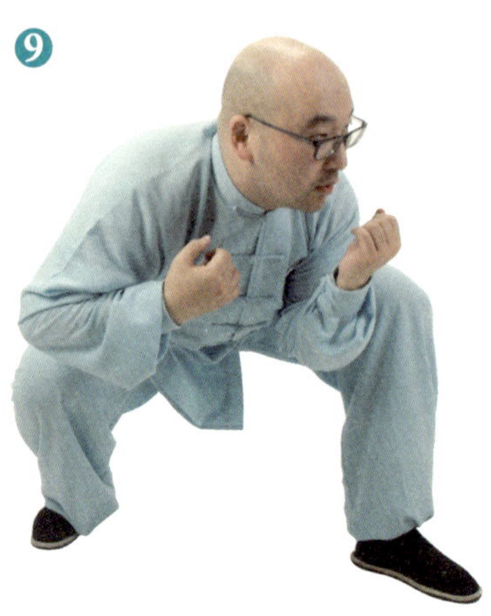

9. Move *qi* like moving a ball, turn inward and downward to shift the body weight to the right foot. Use the hands to press the imaginary ball.

10. Move *qi* like moving a ball 45° upward and forward to shift the body weight to the left foot. Then punch with the fists. Allow your body and footwork to naturally follow the momentum of the punch without forcing any movement.

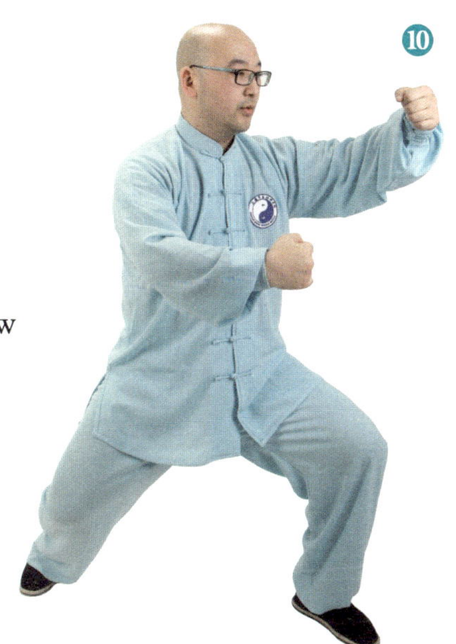

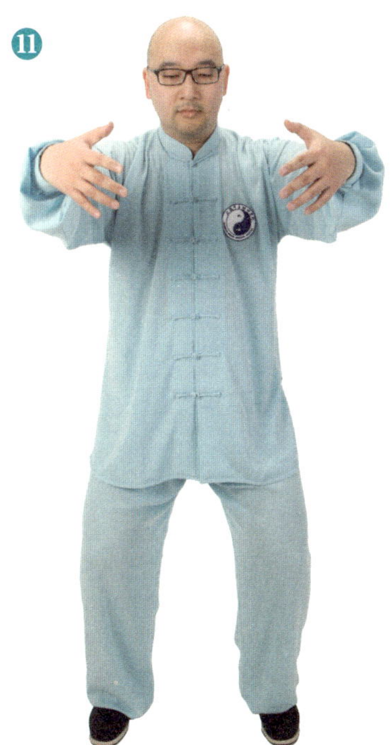

11. Return to standing posture with imagination of holding a ball: Place your feet shoulder-width apart, slightly bend your knees and do not let your knees go past your toes, and raise your arms to the level of your chest.

Movement Eight: Seven Times of Bouncing to Relieve All Diseases

About the movement: This movement focuses on ascending of mental intent and descending of *qi* activity. Rhythmic bouncing of the feet can benefit intervertebral joints and ligaments and help to remove turbid *qi* from Yongquan acupoint (KI 1)[1]. This movement can benefit circulation of cerebrospinal fluid and spinal cord and thus prevent or treat vertebral disorders.

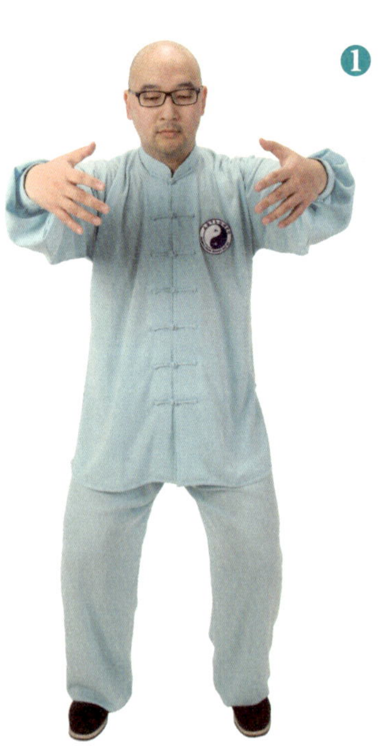

1. Standing posture with imagination of holding a ball: Place your feet shoulder-width apart, slightly bend your knees and do not let your knees go past your toes, and raise your arms to the level of your chest.

---

1 An acupuncture point located on the sole, in the depression appearing on the anterior part of the sole when the foot is in the plantar flexion, approximately at the junction of the anterior third and posterior two-thirds of the line connecting the base of the 2nd and 3rd toes and the heel.

2. Move *qi* like moving a ball to the soles, guiding your body weight and hands to descend slowly.

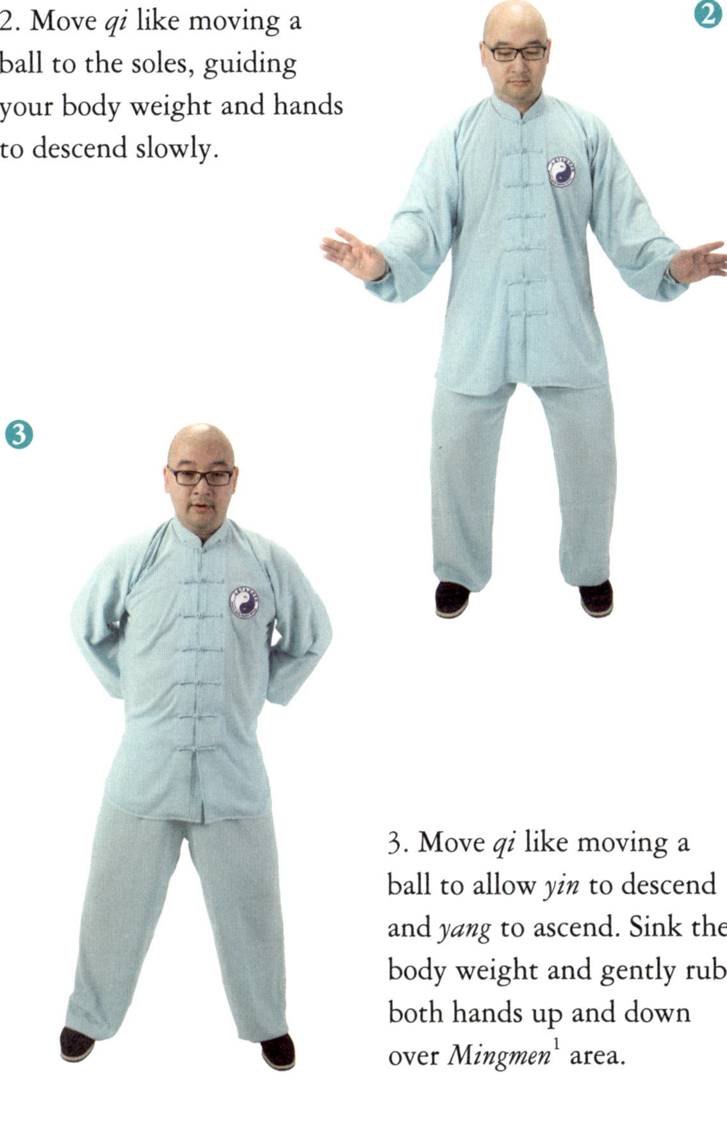

3. Move *qi* like moving a ball to allow *yin* to descend and *yang* to ascend. Sink the body weight and gently rub both hands up and down over *Mingmen*[1] area.

1 *Mingmen* literally means the gate of life, which is located between the kidneys, at the level of the second lumbar vertebrae.

4. Move *qi* like moving a ball to allow *yin* to descend and *yang* to ascend. Follow this with fast bouncing of the feet and dropping of the hands. Then repeat steps 3 to 4 seven times.

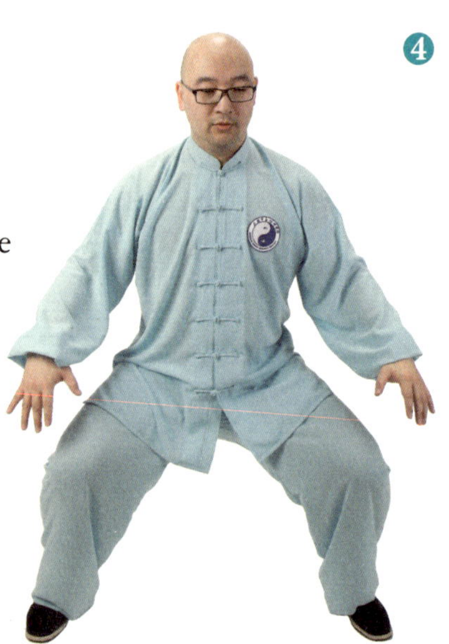

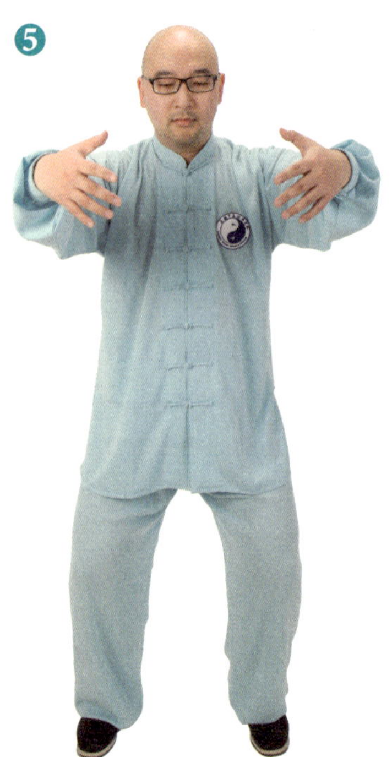

5. Return to standing posture with imagination of holding a ball: Place your feet shoulder-width apart, slightly bend your knees and do not let your knees go past your toes, and raise your arms to the level of your chest.

Chapter Four
Application

Practicing *Ba Duan Jin* is more than a series of physical movements—it is a path toward harmony of body and mind. With consistent and mindful practice, it cultivates the unity of form and spirit, promotes the smooth flow of *qi* and blood, and enhances both mental clarity and physical vitality. *Ba Duan Jin* helps restore balance, prevent illness, and support overall well-being. In the following sections, we will explore its practical benefits and how it can be applied to improve health in daily life.

Multidirectional Regulation

Ba Duan Jin movements help us to achieve tranquility first, then relaxation, and finally smooth circulation of *qi* and blood. Daoists practice *Ba Duan Jin* to resolve *qi* stagnation and blood stasis due to long-term meditation. Martial artists practice *Ba Duan Jin* to stretch the sinews and move *qi* throughout the entire body. Health cultivation advocates practising *Ba Duan Jin* to remove diseases, achieve longevity and cultivate one's moral character. *Ba Duan Jin* can regulate our body and mind in a comprehensive way. It is strongly based on the theory that "when there is sufficient healthy *qi* inside, the pathogenic *qi* have no way to invade the body" and "genuine *qi* will be with you when you achieve *Tian* (peaceful joy), *Dan* (no greed for fame and wealth), *Xu* (void) and *Wu* (nothingness)." Actually, *Ba Duan Jin* practice can change our life attitude and lifestyle and rekindle new energy to experience the subtle beauty of life, just like quotes from the *Zhuang Zi*, *Qi Wu Lun*, "Where there is birth there must be death; where there is death there must be birth. Where there is acceptability there must be unacceptability; where there is unacceptability there must be acceptability."

Disease Prevention and Treatment

If we are equipped with a peaceful mind and sufficient healthy *qi*, we won't get sick. However, it's unlikely to be completely free from worries in the real world. At times, even a brief moment of inner calm, when combined with the guiding movements of *Ba Duan Jin* and specific breathing techniques involving sound, can help address various health conditions. Examples are as follows:

For liver-*qi* stagnation manifesting as chest tightness, irritability, distending pain in the rib-side area, dizziness and tinnitus, practice Movement One and Movement Two on a regular basis.

For spleen deficiency and *qi* stagnation manifesting as abdominal distension and pain, a poor appetite, nausea, vomiting and indigestion, it's advisable to practice Movement Two and Movement Three.

For disharmony between the heart and kidney manifesting as dizziness, tinnitus, insomnia, dream-disturbed sleep, soreness and weakness in the low back and knee joints, feverish sensations in the palms, soles and chest, practice Movement Five and Movement Six.

For failure of clean *yang* to ascend, practice Movement Four and Movement Seven.

For hyperactivity of liver-*yang*, practice Movement Four and Movement Eight.

For cerebro-cardiovascular diseases, practice Movements One to Four.

For respiratory system conditions, practice Movements One to Three and Movement Seven.

For digestive system problems, practice Movement Three and Movement Five.

For neck and low back pain, practice Movements Four to Six.

It's worth noting that many factors need to be taken into consideration. These may include *yin*, *yang*, deficiency, excess, exterior, interior, cold, heat, individualized constitution, geographical locations and seasons.

Appendix
The Meridian Charts

For reference, the following diagram—originating from ancient Chinese medical texts—illustrates the main twelve meridians, the Conception and Governor Vessels, and their associated acupoints, as well as the Thoroughfare and Belt Vessels mentioned in the text.

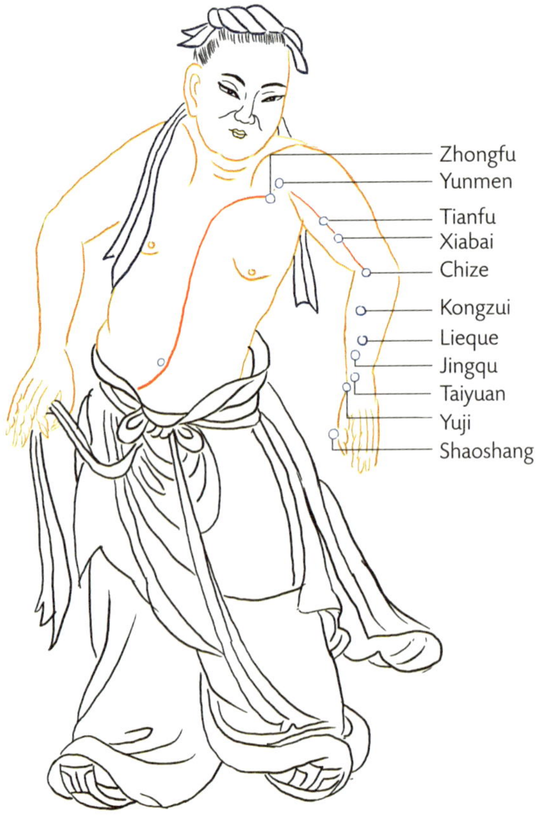

Taiyin Lung Meridian of the Hand (LU)

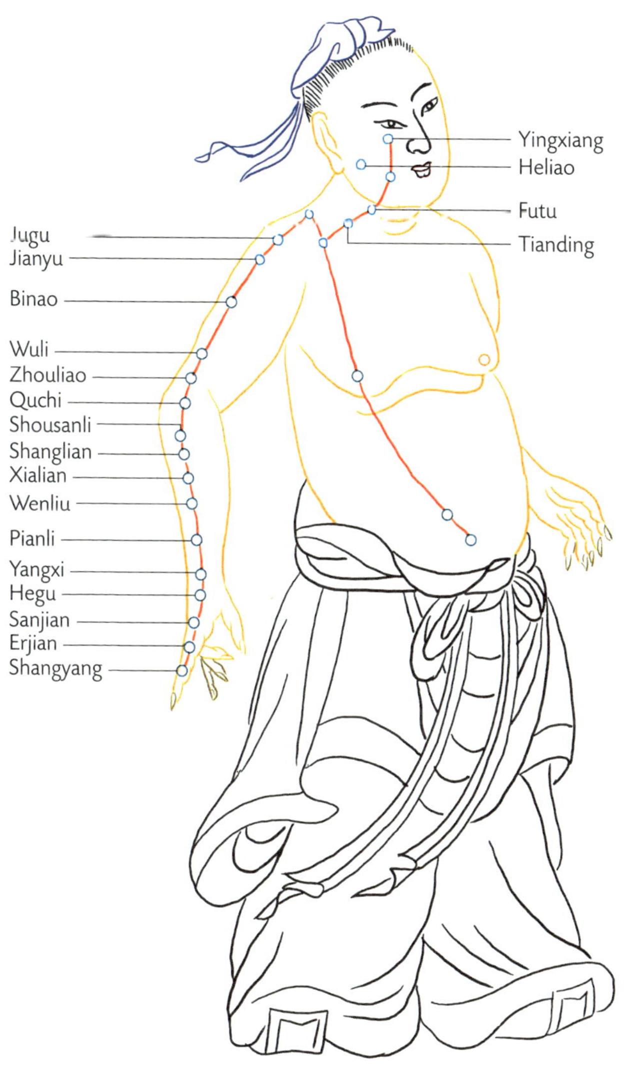

Yangming Large Intestine Meridian of the Hand (LI)

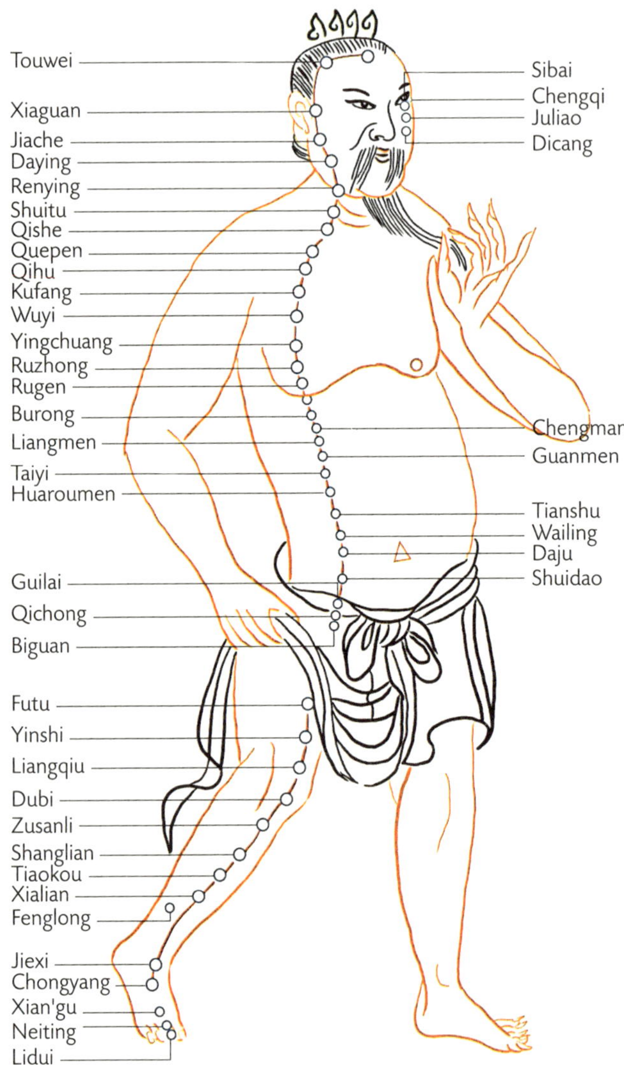

Yangming Stomach Meridian of the Foot (ST)

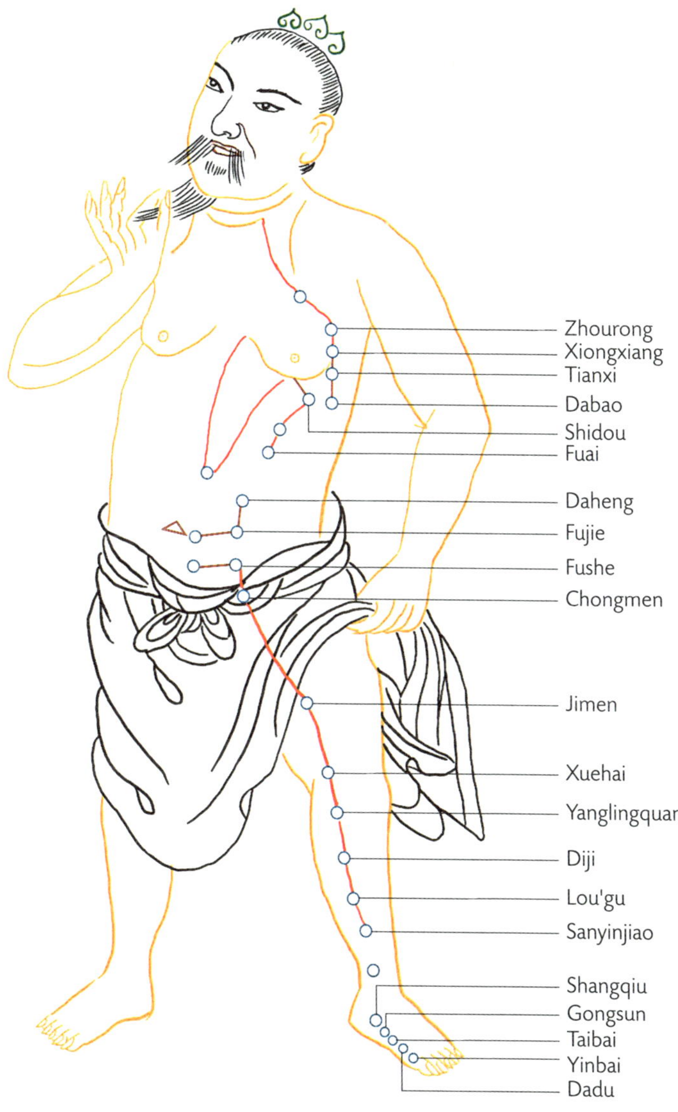

Taiyin Spleen Meridian of the Foot (SP)

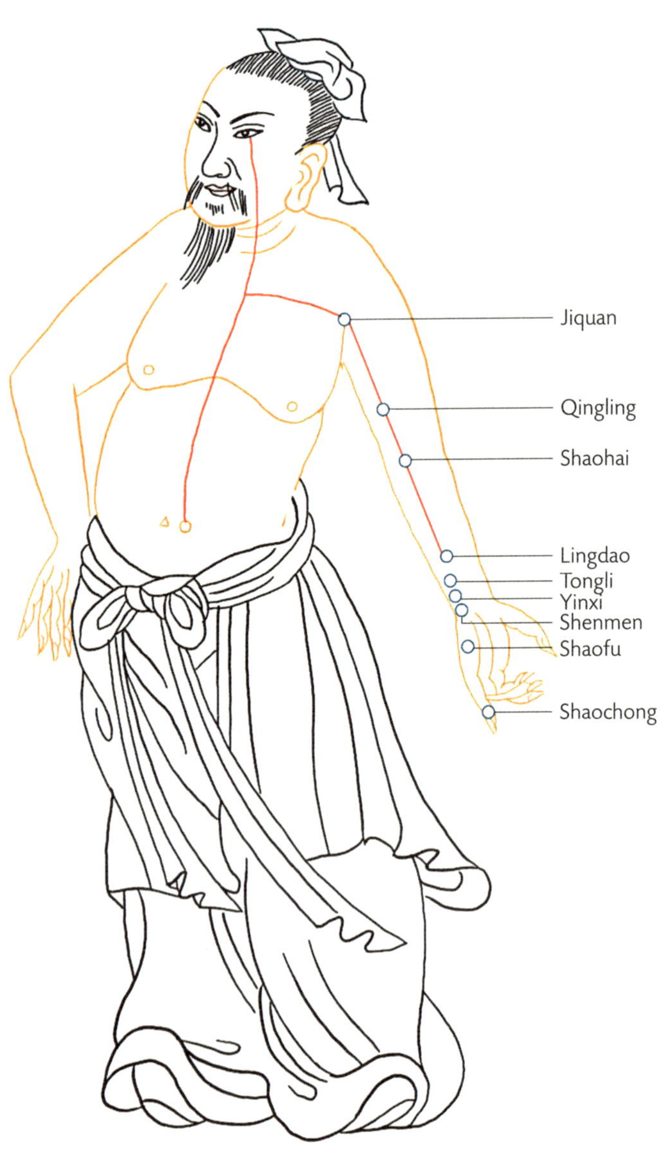

Shaoyin Heart Meridian of the Hand (HT)

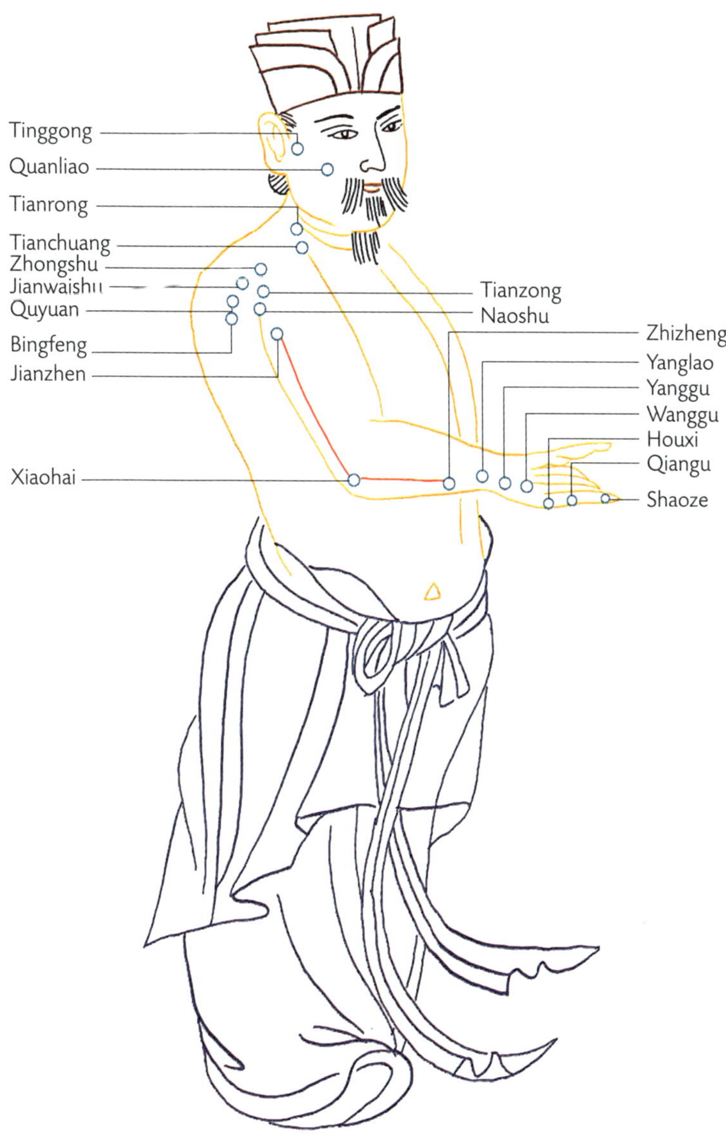

Taiyang Small Intestine Meridian of the Hand (SI)

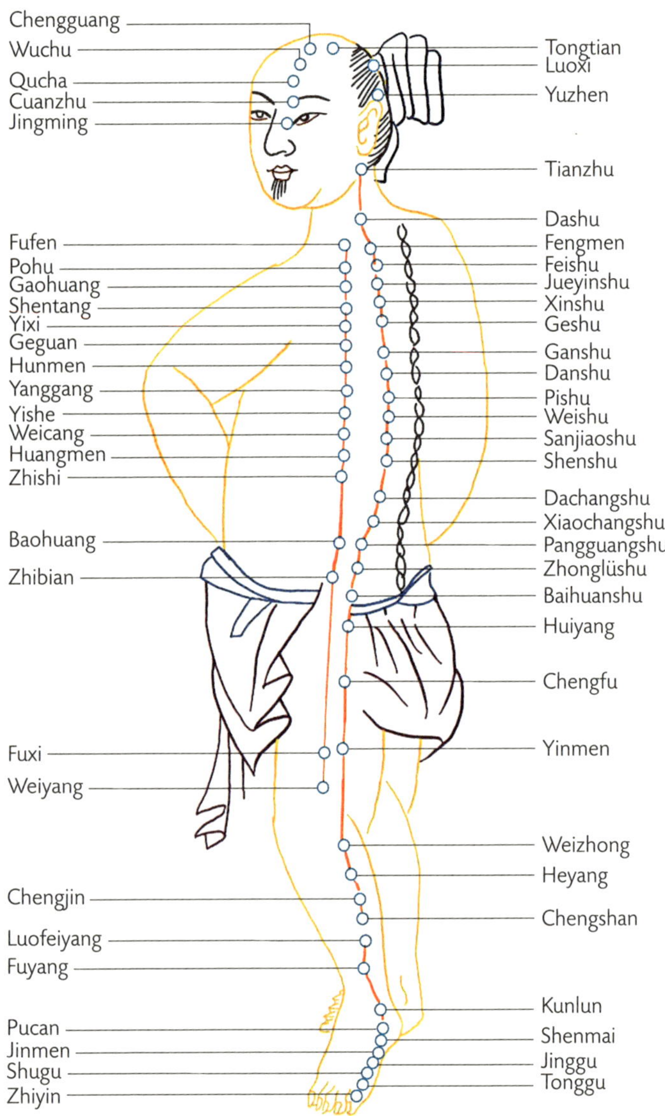

Taiyang Bladder Meridian of the Foot (BL)

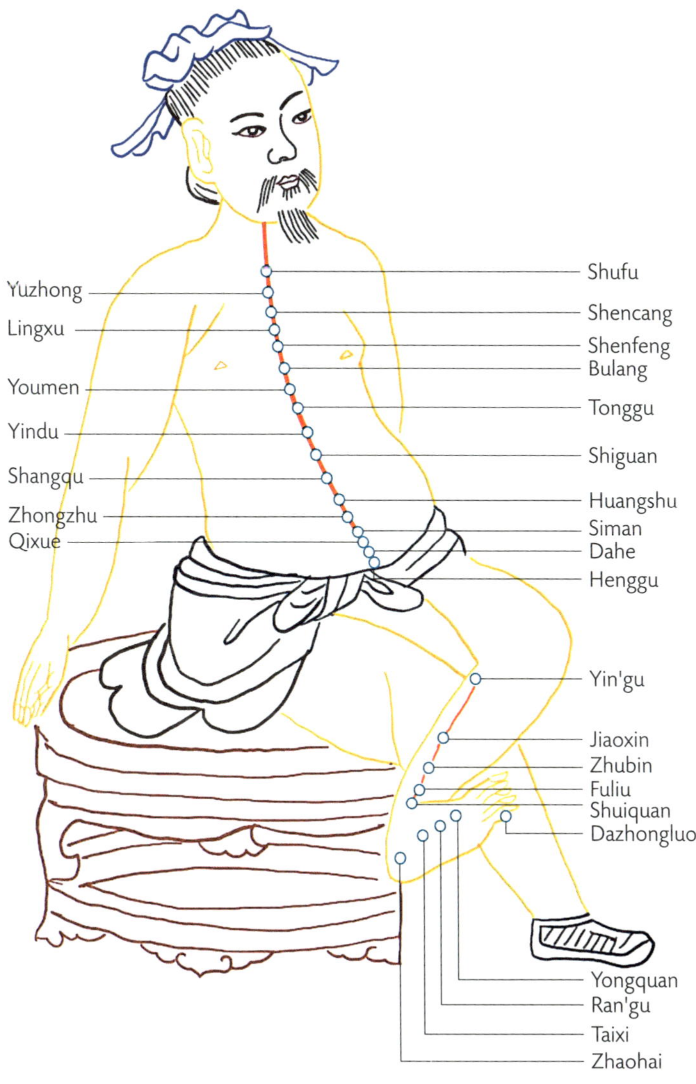

Shaoyin Kidney Meridian of the Foot (KI)

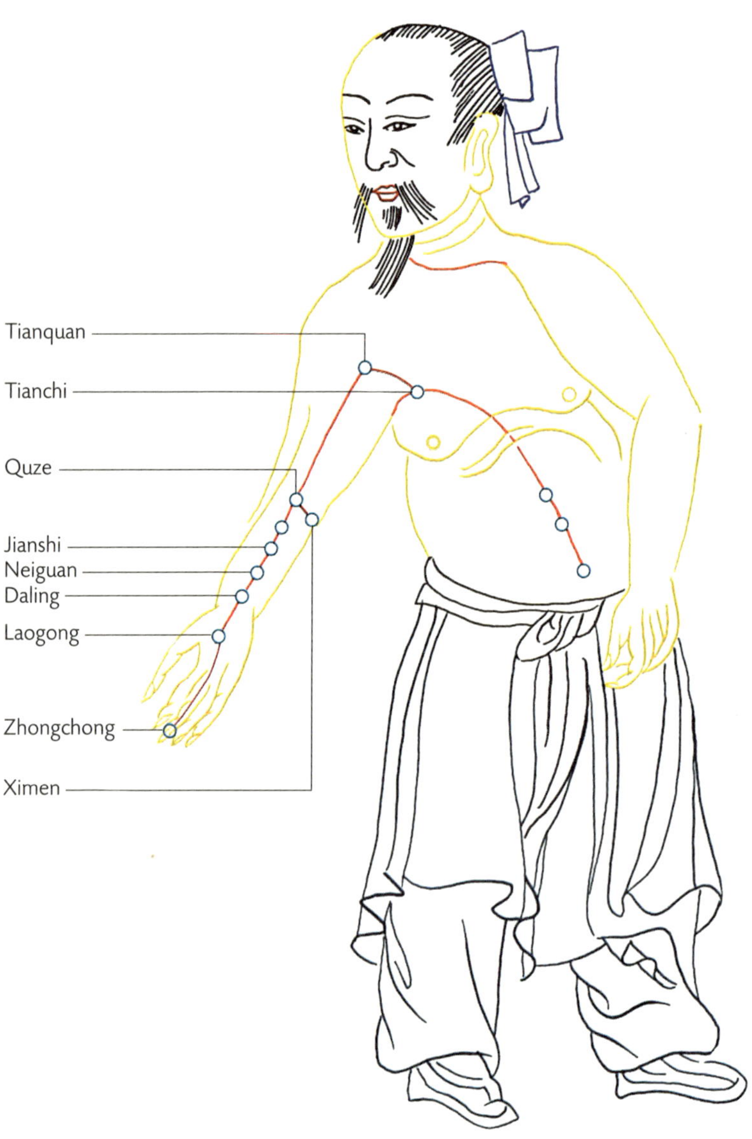

Jueyin Pericardium Meridian of the Hand (PC)

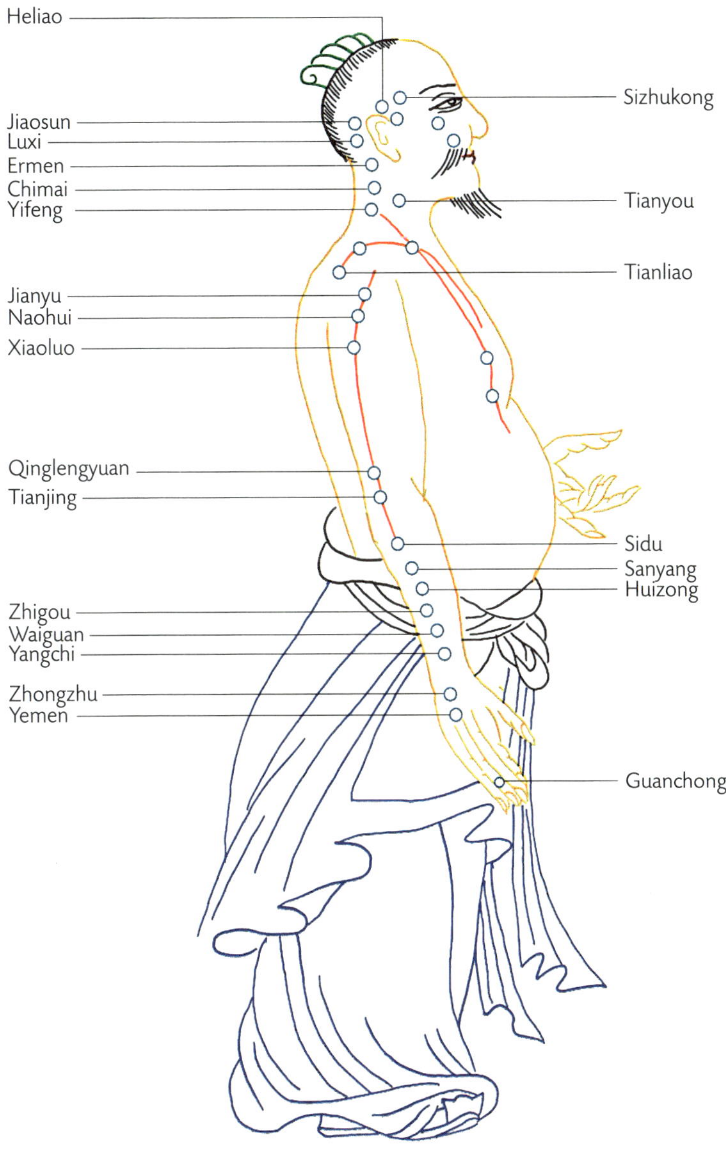

Shaoyang Triple Energizer (*Sanjiao*) Meridian of the Hand (TE)

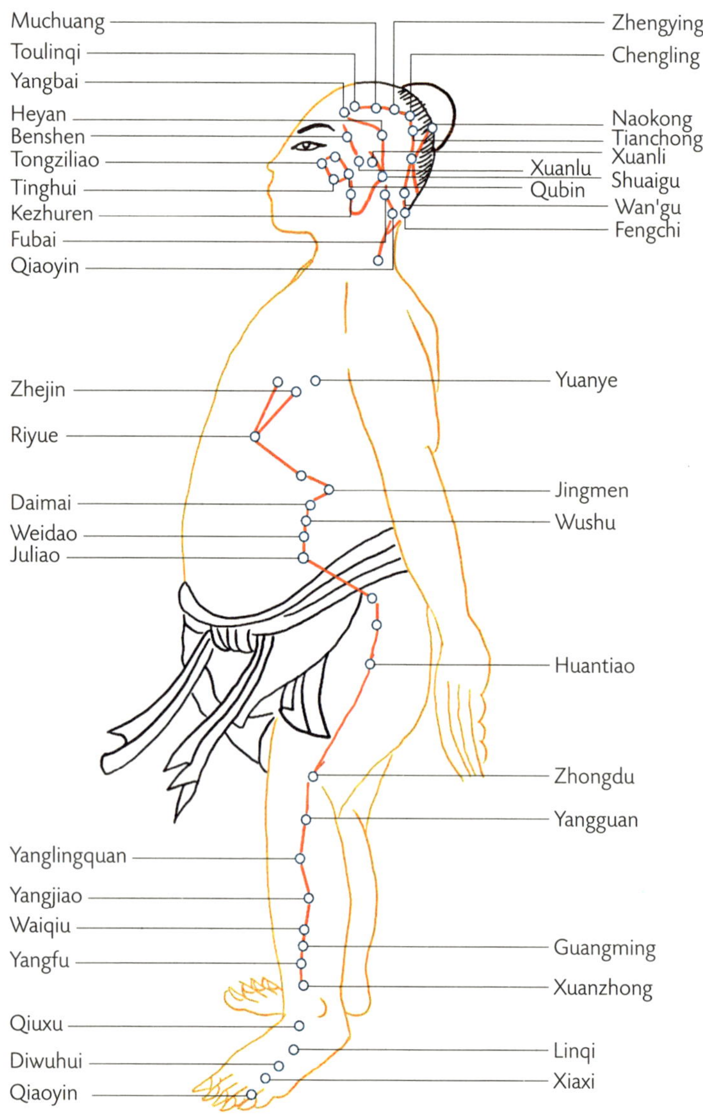

Shaoyang Gallbladder Meridian of the Foot (GB)

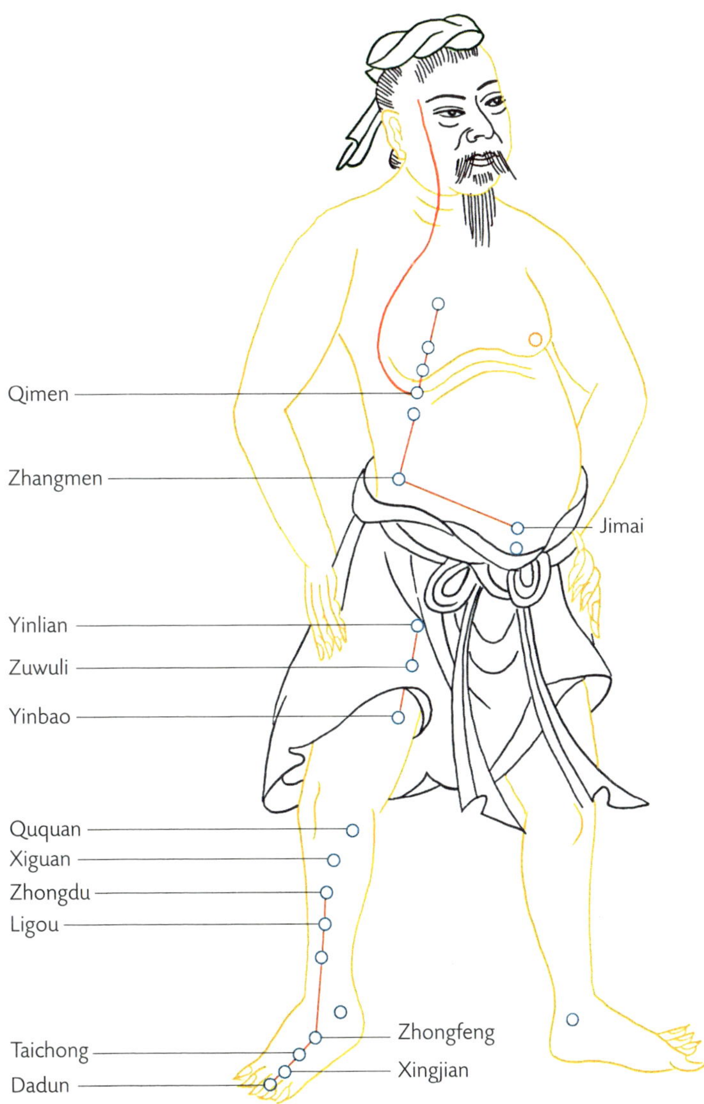

Jueyin Liver Meridian of the Foot (LR)

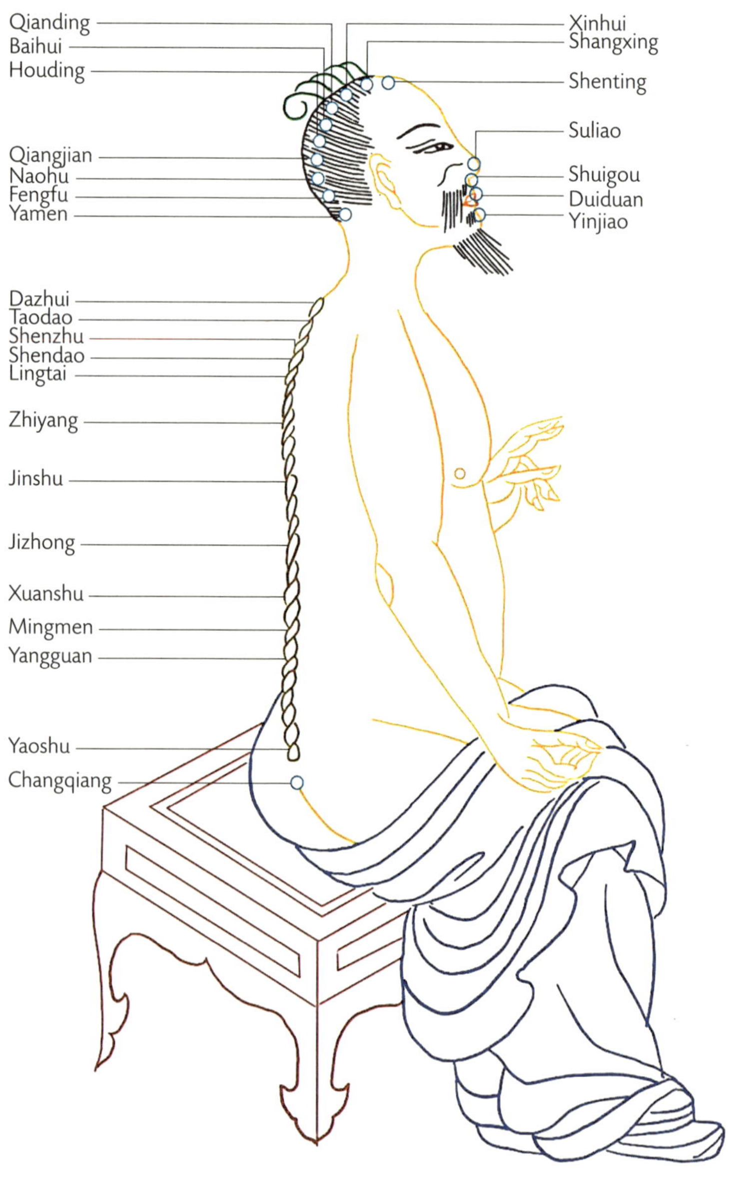

Governor Vessel (GV)

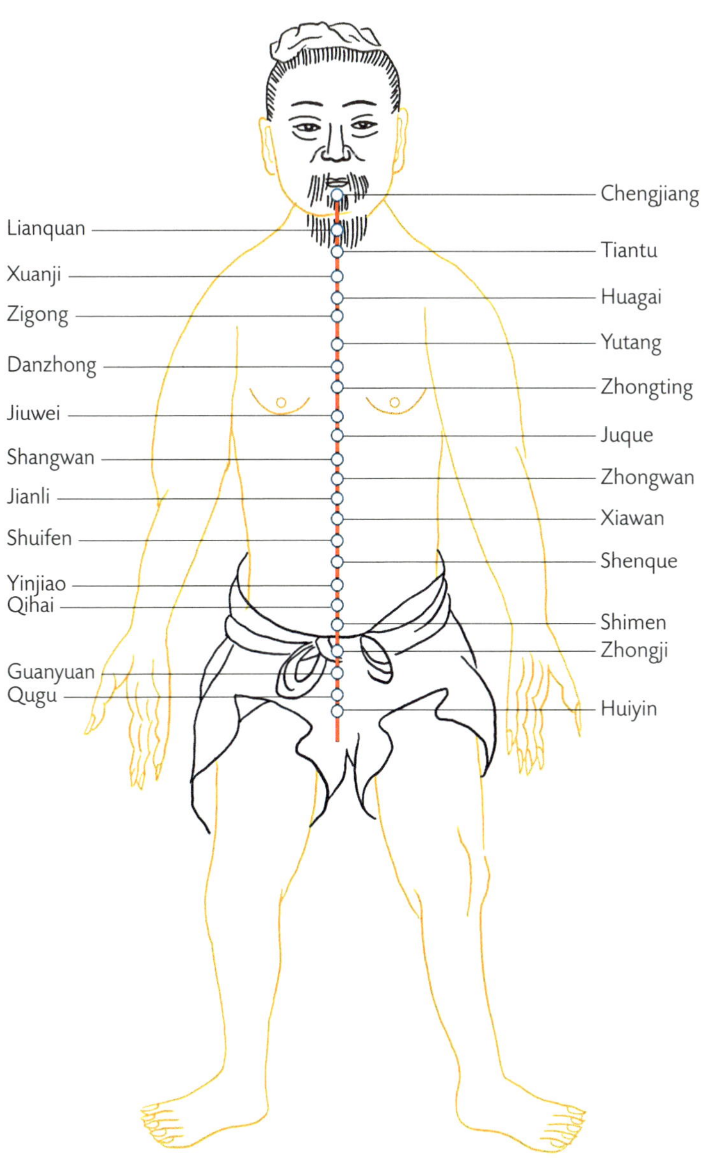

Conception Vessel (CV)

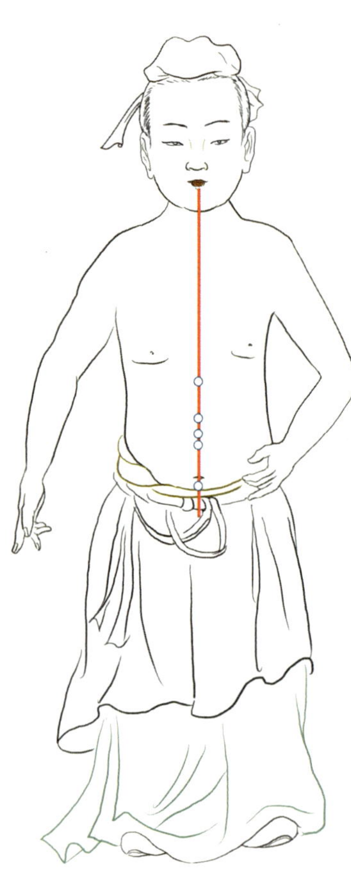

Thoroughfare Vessel (Chong)

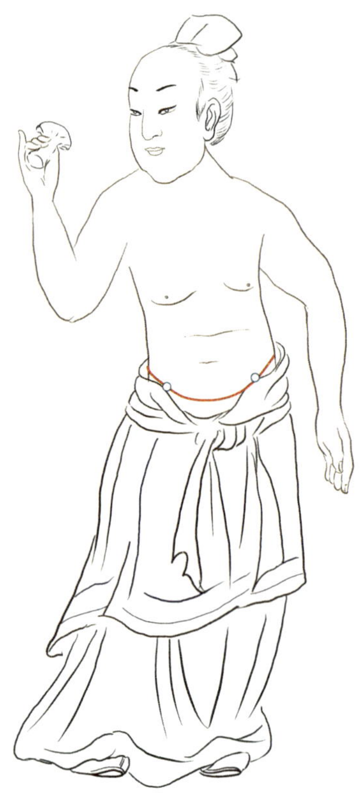

Belt Vessel (Dai)